STRENGTH to STAND

Surviving Guillain-Barré and Pulling Back the Curtain on Long-Term Care

Copyright © 2025 by Sonja Stukel Schmieder

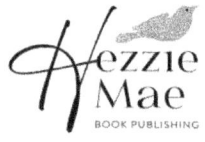
REL Print Group, a Hezzie Mae Publication
Duluth, MN.
www.HezzieMae.com

All rights reserved. Hezzie Mae supports copyright. Copyright fuels creativity, encourages diverse voices, promotes free speech, and creates a vibrant culture. Thank you for complying with copyright laws by not reproducing, scanning, or distributing any part of this book in any form without permission from the publisher.

ISBN: 979-8-9911532-6-3

Cover Design: Hailee Pavey @paveydesign.com
Cover Inspiration: Linda Bjorkland

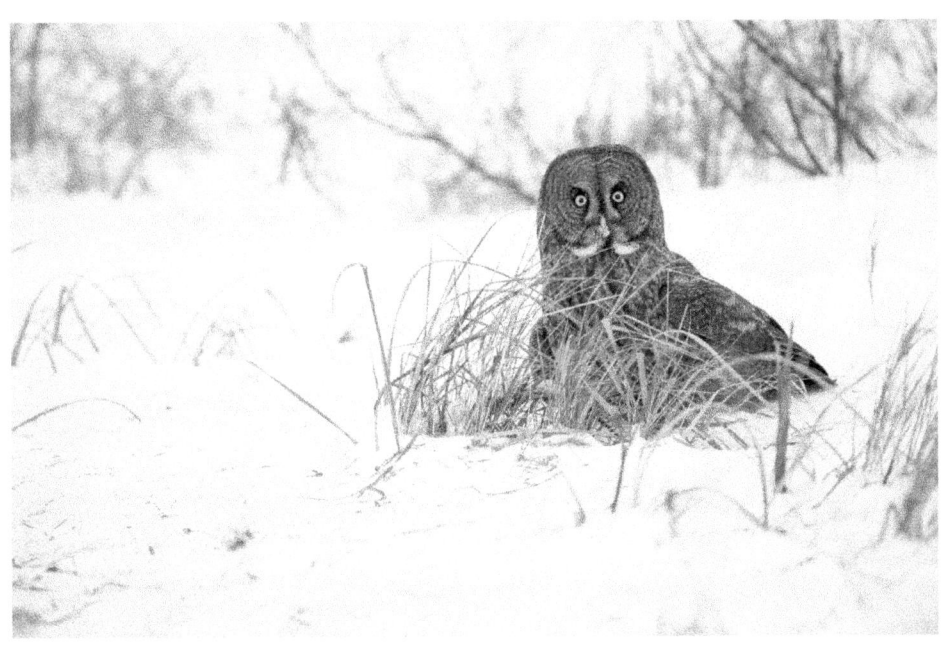

Gene Stukel Photography
Granite Falls, Minnesota

STRENGTH to STAND

Surviving Guillain-Barré and
Pulling Back the Curtain on Long-Term Care

Sonja Stukel Schmieder

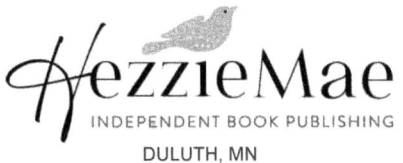

HezzieMae
INDEPENDENT BOOK PUBLISHING
DULUTH, MN

Dedication

To my daughter, my heart, my everything, Lily, who had an older mommy and never made me feel old, and who never, ever "lets go my hand."

And to all those whose lives have been diminished by illness and old age, who now reside in long-term care in Skilled Nursing Facilities, and to their caregivers.

It is dedicated to my mom and dad, Matt and Gert, who always moved with the times and never dwelled on age. Their gatherings included everyone, regardless of age. They loved life no matter how difficult and fought to the end—with grit and no excuses—to keep on living.

Acknowledgements

The acknowledgements section is usually found at the end of a book. However, I could not, in good conscience, relegate this section there. The names of those who unfailingly offered encouragement and far-sightedness in my quest to tell my story, need to be listed at the front. I am so grateful to each of these individuals. My love is right back at you!

Great thanks and love to Gene and Helen, Jim and Mary, my caring and attentive brothers and sisters-in-law, my constant cheerleaders – through sickness to better health – who were faithful first-readers of the bits and pieces that miraculously became a book. Their collective insights into a more suitable book title were ingenious.

I appreciate Tom and Bob, readers, helpers, and forever friends. I also want to thank Martha, my most perfect person. We go back thirty-some years to our Washington, DC, days; she always knows the right words to comfort, quiet, and soothe. Like me, she comes from good people. Martha created the book's digital files, copying and pasting all text. Great thanks to Greg, who lives miles from here but is never very far away.

I am fortunate to have longtime friends Carol, Gretchen, and Linda in my life. When I need "a helping hand," they are always there for me, with goodies and laughter! Our conversations are priceless. Shoutout to Gretchen for occasional visits while her spouse was also in a long-term care facility. To Carol for keeping up-to-date on my progress. And to Linda for our many exchanges about the book.

To teachers: In appreciation of your extraordinary efforts to educate and instruct students by breaking down new and often complex information, concepts, and abstractions into understandable language, enabling them to learn, experience the joy of learning, and recognize their capabilities.

Brad is a constant in my life. If I had had a say in choosing a son-in-law, he would have received my vote, hands down! This remarkable man always steps up to the plate.

To my grandchildren, Leon and Lera: I love you zillions and long for the days ahead when we can run and play together again. Rubio and Mimi, little dogs extraordinaire, I wish to grow even older with you both by my side.

I am deeply grateful to University of Minnesota physicians, Matthew A. Hunt, MD, my neurosurgeon, and Gautam G. Jha, MD, my oncologist, who have been quietly adamant that I still have "miles to go..." (Robert Frost). Great appreciation to Arun Idiculla, MD, a physical and rehabilitation physician at Courage Kenny Rehabilitation Institute, for finding ways to to get me "on the move!"

Finally, my great thanks to Heather, my publisher and new friend, for her skill and expertise in advancing the book along so quickly. And thank you for making the experience so much fun! For Heather, the author and the author's vision and words are on equal footing. Our friendship will go beyond this time and space.

"Nothing ever becomes real until it is experienced."
John Keats

Foreword

More than thirty years ago, Sonja and I worked together in a biotech company in Maryland. Her vivacity was contagious. She lit up any room just by entering it. Her entrance into the world of disabilities because of Guillain-Barré Syndrome was a jolt to anyone who had known her and a sobering reality check for all of us that sudden, debilitating changes are always a possibility.

The world of medicine has long been the source of novels, television shows, and movies, but nearly always from the viewpoint of the clinicians. What Sonja does with this book is to turn the table and tell the story from the perspective of the consumer rather than the producer. Few have attempted such a task. Her insights will be a guide for those of us who become consumers of skilled nursing, as well as for its producers, who too often keep a distance from their consumers to the detriment of both.

Gregory A. Prince, DDS, PhD

TABLE OF CONTENTS

Section 1
Imaginings: A Changed Life 1

Section 2
The Site: A Skilled Nursing Facility 9

Section 3
The Residents: The Centerpiece of Any Facility 37
The Nursing Staff, the Heart of Any Facility 72

Section 4
Management: Orchestrating Care 93

Section 5
Leadership in Action 151

Gaining an Understanding 169
Resources and References 171
About The Author 173

Dear Reader,

For years, I was the caregiver, and then suddenly found that I was the one who needed care. My health had declined, and I had contracted a disabling condition. I began to feel the effects of aging.

We all age, and as we do, we may need care and support beyond what our families and friends can provide.

This mini-book of mini-chapters, snippets of information, randomings, and simple observations is written to provide a first-hand account of life in a Skilled Nursing Facility (SNF), the name frequently used to replace the term "nursing home."

The book focuses on the lives of the aged and sick who reside within such facilities, particularly those in long-term care.

It is one viewpoint about a single SNF to enlighten the following audiences: those who are already part of or wish to join an SNF caregiving team, those considering what their future path might hold, those involved in seeking more intensive care for someone in need; those from other generations who find joy in interacting with seniors and their families; those in positions of authority tasked with making prudent decisions about our sick and aging population; those who recognize the value of working with an aging population that continues to grow; and those who simply find fulfillment in helping others.

It presents sketches or glimpses of daily life within such facilities, including the people involved, their challenges, and their cheerleaders.

It provides basic information about SNFs you might not know or have thought much about; it touches upon core program components of SNFs and how their leadership addresses them.

It is not just a story about the strength and resilience of long-term residents; it is an expanded and detailed description of how one SNF housing these residents operates and conducts business. It calls for closer scrutiny of the inner workings of such facilities and serves as a call to action for greater support and better treatment of this population. It also asks for more stories from more facilities.

It recognizes the good efforts in managing such facilities and seeks an even higher level of excellence.

Some assume that all who reside at an SNF are ancient, weak, and too sick to recover. Others assume every resident has dementia or Alzheimer's. While some long-term residents fit those descriptors, some individuals recover and require only temporary but extensive care that families simply cannot manage themselves. For these residents, it is a place of planned care and support that encourages (and gently demands) resident improvement and advancement.

My story fights against the assumption that long-term care residents have no hopes or dreams left and are merely sad, alone, and forgotten.

Additionally, it is meant to erase the perception that long-term care at a SNF is only an end-of-the-road stop. It seeks to dispel the notion that there is no return to normalcy once a resident of such a facility moves on.

It broadens the definition of care and support for the sick and elderly, shifting from a TLC perspective (tender loving care by the nurses) to one that includes the ramifications of management decisions regarding these residents. It emphasizes how both factors affect the health and well-being of long-term residents, who, in addition to striving to improve their physical health, are also forced to concentrate their energies on solving everyday concerns and problems.

It further describes my medical condition—Guillain-Barré Syndrome—to help raise awareness of this rapid-onset, slow-to-recover debilitating disorder and spark new avenues of research in its prevention and treatment.

The book is my way of stepping up as a happy warrior, "a constant influence," as William Wordsworth put it, for the elderly, the sick, the infirm, the unwell, the unsteady, the disabled, the weak, and the frail. I share my story with those who have triumphed to live another day!

My story may be similar to that of others who reside in SNFs, or it might not be. The workings of this particular facility may or may not be commonplace. I can only share what I've experienced. But when one has a story to tell, it must be told! The words come easily, and there are many of them. So, this is my story—a true account of my life over the past two years in long-term care at a Skilled Nursing Facility, confronting the challenges of sickness and aging and the issues and problems that arise in SNFs.

The fact that a resident would write about life in a Skilled Nursing Facility is notable; sharing my experiences "on the inside" has become my mission.

Writing the book presented its challenges. When I began, my fingers slid across the keyboard too easily, leading to frequent errors. However, I discovered I could text and input information word by word. My old iPhone 6 came through, even though it overheated at times.

My daughter had mentioned to me more than once, "Mom, you almost died four times," prompting me to ask God again and again, "Why did you spare me? For what purpose?" This book was the answer—it needed to be written.

I sincerely hope that it will be a resource for you. As you read the book, take a breather now and then. Share with anyone who might be helped by its contents.

Sonja

1

Imaginings: A Changed Life

Many years ago, a famous someone named John Lennon wrote a song called "Imagine." A line from the song says, "All the people livin' for today." This was interpreted to mean "all the people as one, living in peace, together."

But I ask, "Might he have meant 'all the people livin' JUST for today? Going on with their lives thinking things will always be as they are now? Oblivious to anything of importance getting in the way of their routines, their take-for-grantedness?'"

I think so, and I will interpret that line in a way that makes us want to appreciate each day to the fullest. Things will not remain the same. Life can change on a dime, and we must appreciate all we have when we have it!

Imagine that, seemingly overnight, you can no longer walk, work, go to church, drive a car, exercise, travel to faraway places, have lunch with friends, grocery shop, go to the Activities Center, or play the piano.

Imagine that you cannot hug your children or cuddle with your grandchildren. Imagine no family outings that include your presence. Imagine the puppies you left behind are now grown and no longer missing you. Imagine only a few calls or visits from friends or work buddies (after all, you live in a "nursing home"); imagine no one asks your opinion about almost anything. (Family gets a huge pass here, as they are in close contact through visits, calls, emails, texts, and FaceTime).

Imagine an initial pain so severe you cannot stand for someone to move you into a more comfortable position in bed, even using soft pillows to keep you stable and in place.

Imagine that controlling the pain will take months.

Imagine a life prolonged by IVs, shots, and pills and defined by MRI and CT-scan images and visits to specialists and family doctors.

Imagine always having to wear a diaper or briefs. The humility!

Imagine having to push a call light for help.

Imagine being bedridden and hearing the fire alarm go off!

Imagine that you initially cannot hold a fork or spoon but can sit up in your bed just enough so that when someone comes along, they will reposition you, put a bib on you, and then feed you at breakfast, lunch, and dinner.

Imaginings: A Changed Life

Imagine being very sick and having to wear a huge, washed-out, faded hospital gown instead of regular clothes or jammies every day and night. Forget looking even somewhat fashionable!

Imagine that you cannot brush your teeth, brush your hair, or trim your nails. Imagine needing help to do your laundry.

Imagine living with a stranger and relearning what it means to share space while respecting the needs and priorities of someone you might not have chosen as a roommate.

Imagine you cannot get your hair cut or colored because you cannot easily travel, cannot put on makeup very well (yikes!), cannot put on your pants or socks by yourself, cannot slip into comfy shoes, or even wear shoes at all. Imagine you cannot stand in front of the bathroom mirror or a full-length mirror to catch even a glimpse of your upright body.

Imagine that you are so sick you don't even care!

Imagine that your spouse has died, and you must face your illness without your partner's love and support. Imagine that you no longer cry about that or about most things.

Imagine that all your belongings have been stored, and you don't have your most precious things around you to comfort you.

Imagine that your medical condition has had a profound effect on your children and has caused an enormous upheaval in their lives as they grapple with your illness, the financial nightmare it brings, and a myriad of inconveniences caused by you not being able to manage your own life. All of this, while at the same time raising very young children—with all that it requires—and working full-time at their respective careers.

> *"I took a deep breath and listened to the old bray of my heart, I am, I am, I am..."*
> Sylvia Plath

A Health Condition: Guillain-Barré Syndrome (GBS)

I don't have to imagine these things...I have lived them.

These imaginings are all effects of Guillain-Barré. Imagine such a condition! It is what I suffer from and why I reside in a Skilled Nursing Facility.

Its formal name is Guillain-Barré Syndrome (Gee-yan Bah-ray), after Guillain and Barré, two French neurologists who first described the condition in 1916. (It's a fancy-sounding name for a terrible disorder.)

Mayo Clinic. (n.d.). Guillain-Barré Syndrome (GBS) is a neurological condition in which the immune system attacks the nerves, causing muscle weakness, numbness, tingling, and extreme fatigue. It is a rare condition, with 3,000–6,000 cases in the U.S. annually.

Experts disagree about the cause of GBS. Some believe it occurs after a viral or bacterial infection. It is not contagious or inherited; it is not curable.

A vast majority of those afflicted recover motor strength within a year. Over time, rehabilitation services and programs are needed to help relieve symptoms and improve flexibility and movement.

GBS: Funding for Research

The National Institute of Health (NIH) funds research on disorders like GBS through one of its 27 institutes, the National Institute of Allergy and Infectious Diseases (NIAID).

I ask that NIAID prioritizes funding for GBS research, studies, and clinical trials to develop a myriad of strategies, interventions, and treatments to address this rare condition. I, too, want to be a strong advocate for GBS awareness, research, and funding.

A Possible Source of Hope: Courage Kenny Rehabilitation Institute

Courage Kenny Rehabilitation Institute (CKRI), from now on referred to as CK, has many sites in Minnesota. Its Golden Valley location, for example, specializes in treating patients with neuro-conditions. CK was established in 2013, merging Sister Kenny Institute and Courage Center; it is part of the Allina Health system. CK seeks to provide "exceptional rehabilitative services" for adults and children with "injuries and disabilities of all kinds."

Trying to Get Into Courage Kenny

My family spoke with CK representatives more than two years ago, in-between hospital stays and short stays at several other Skilled Nursing Facilities, to see if I might be accepted there for rehabilitation. CK is renowned for its work with GBS patients.

Its therapists are experts in the best and most up-to-date treatments and apparatuses that help restore physical functions so patients can return to acceptable daily living.

My family members were asked at the time if they thought I could handle a comprehensive rehabilitation program occurring several days a week for perhaps hours each day. Given my inability to move without pain, the reality of attending CK seemed premature and even ridiculous at the time. Better to get the pain under control, try to regain some mobility, and then transfer to CK at a later date when I could withstand a more rigorous regimen of physical and occupational therapies.

My Last Hospital Stay

The last hospital where I was confined for a couple of weeks gave me 24 hours notice before they would need to release me. The social workers at the hospital began to seek yet another Skilled Nursing Facility where I might reside.

Negotiations between this Skilled Nursing Facility and the hospital occurred without my family's involvement. Please note: Lily, Jim, and Carol did everything they could to find the most accommodating facility for my needs during the first seven months of GBS. We were not familiar with this facility, including how it would manage my GBS. My children were out of town but were told that only one bed was available in the Twin Cities at this particular facility in long-term care, but not transitional care, as requested.

Imaginings: A Changed Life

The facility needed a deposit of $6,000 the next day to hold the room. We secured the room almost under duress and thought of it only as another point in my care journey. And so, this is why I came to live at this facility.

Strength to Stand

2

The Site:
A Skilled Nursing Facility

You Live Where? Many families and friends are living or have lived the following scenario:

"Why can't I go to Gramma's house?" he asked.
"Gramma doesn't live there anymore," said his mother.
"I want to see Gramma!!" he vehemently responded.

Let's step back a bit. Gramma suddenly got very sick and needed to be in a safe, supportive, and healthy environment where her care could be managed and monitored. This meant she would have to leave her home and move to a more suitable place- one that exists for just this kind of script.

The dialogue goes something like this:

"We can't possibly care for her in our home. Where will she go? How do we find a good place for her?"

This is the thought process:

"I can't bear to think of her in: 1) an old folks' home or nursing home, one bereft of cool, with-it, fully-functioning people and happenings; 2) a place of skinny, frail bodies sitting in wheelchairs, wrapped in sweaters or soft blankets, or bent over walkers on their way down the hall; 3) a "home" that is way too quiet, even at mealtimes, where time passes so slowly you can hear the tick-tick-tick of the clock, and where boredom reigns!"

Let's explore and get rid of some concerns expressed in that storyline and move on to the reality of life in a Skilled Nursing Facility.

This Skilled Nursing Facility

I live in an old, nondescript building on the corner of a busy street in the heart of a big and wonderful city. Adjacent to the site, billed as a health and rehabilitation center, is a parking lot with spaces for staff and guests.

The first floor has a comforting, neutral-colored entryway and a comfortable sitting area with a kitchenette next to the patio. It also houses offices for Management, rooms for short-stay residents, and the Chapel—complete with a grand piano—for believers and peace-seekers.

The lower level houses the physical and occupational therapy room and equipment, a few meeting rooms, and rooms for doctors' screenings and exams. It also includes a daycare. Floors two and three accommodate around 100 residents in private or semi-private rooms. There, too, are nurses' stations, dining areas, more offices, and small living rooms for guests.

The Site: A Skilled Nursing Facility

The facility provides short-term care for residents transitioning from hospital to home and long-term care "for people who require 24-hour skilled nursing care for advanced health needs."

All care here "is based on the belief that mind, body, and spirit are intricately connected." The site's unique focus is providing spiritual care to its residents. Spiritual care includes Protestant and Catholic worship services in the Chapel, Hymn singing, Bible studies, and Communion, as well as activities designed to comfort residents.

Pastor John is a shy, quiet man whose motto is to serve the needs of residents through the powers of faith and music. This pastor's definition of service extends to assisting with the workings of the facility in any way he can. For example, the other day, he grabbed a tool case and tried to fix my leg braces when the locks refused to work. Catch Pastor John's morning breakfast blast at 8:40 AM over the PA System. His positive messages are sent to residents and staff to welcome a new and promising day.

Mary Ann is the Associate Pastor. Her kindness and compassion for others and her love for her family are evident.

A Unique Feature

Grandma's House Children's Center is the facility's employer-sponsored daycare program for up to 14 of the neighborhood's children. The founder, Mary Ann, initially envisioned a place where children would learn not to fear residents within the facility because of their "wheelchairs, walkers, and wrinkles" and grow to find joy in interacting with them. The hope was that these children would transfer their acceptance of the residents they interact with to the disabled and elderly in the outside world!

The Food

Facilities like this one are pretty adamant about residents getting their nutrients every day, as chronic conditions like diabetes, cancer, and Alzheimer's can cause them to become malnourished. Kitchen staff work hard to prepare healthy meals—three per day—for over 100 residents. This can be a challenge. As we all know, not everyone in any household likes the same foods! The nutritionist must also know residents' special dietary orders and preferences.

Here, we get the usual filler-uppers: pasta and pasta salad, a slice of bread, rice, potatoes, a fruit bowl, a piece of often tough meat, and a soft and mushy, pudding-like dessert. If we are lucky, we get BLTs.

A hint: Just in case a resident refuses "to eat that again," request that a family member or friend brings a sack of snacks for those days when nothing on the menu appeals. (Food services offer a request-your-own meal available through a phone-in number that includes an array of options.) Besides, the occasional bag of chips or mini-Snickers bars can do wonders to lift one's spirits; enough said!

Remember when food was made and served with love? I long for even a hint of those bygone days.

Housekeeping

Our primary housekeeper, Sweet Teresa, is tiny but effortlessly handles the Mop & Glo, a heavy machine. Brenda is always cheerful and accommodating.

Laundry

Most facilities offer laundry services to residents on-site. The washing and drying of clothes, which includes putting individual items on hangers, is no small responsibility for the laundry service staff. Wanda is the facility's leading laundry lady with two friendly assistants. They're responsible for wardrobe oversight for over 100 residents. Wanda goes out of her way to find any missing or unlabeled items. She helpfully suggests we request reimbursement for any items that may have been ruined or completely disappeared.

Scents and Sounds

The scents wafting throughout an SNF can be intense at times and are a mix of those that are acceptable and those that are not.

Pungent smells can add another dimension of stuffiness to an already locked-down facility. These are, however, deliberately offset by the sweet, rich fragrance of fresh flowers like roses and lilacs (which also add color and beauty to any room). Room sprays help the cause, too.

Sachets of lavender or vanilla line our cabinet drawers, and whiffs of someone's sweet perfume are caught on the fly.

Our housekeepers leave us a scented, scrubbed, mean, and clean floor.

The aromas of many different kinds of food from restaurants in the neighborhood, the strong and glorious smell of coffee brewing, and exhaust fumes from buses and cars, all unchecked, are now a familiar and comforting part of living at this site.

Our meal trays often contain strawberries, raspberries, and a garlic roll, each containing another familiar scent.

I miss the smell of freshly mown grass and the best of all scents: fresh, cool, crisp air coming through the window of our room, making the window curtains dance!

What can we hear? We hear soft or loud sounds; we hear music, the sweet sound of music. Sounds awaken us and demand that we come alive!

Through our open windows, we hear the frequent roar of cars, delivery trucks, motorcycles, and city buses, police and emergency vehicle sirens, dogs barking, cicadas, bees, owls, and chirping birds, rain and thunder, the wind, and nightlife.

Inside, we hear the soft footsteps of the nurses on duty, one of them calling my name; agitated cries from an uncomfortable resident; intercom messages; the beep-beep of healthcare machines; favorite songs being YouTubed; residents' TVs tuned into the news, game shows, soaps, sports, or classic movies; and the tick-tick-tick of my clock.

The Site: A Skilled Nursing Facility

On the Go

Everywhere there is construction and bumper-to-bumper traffic. No big deal, for I am out in the world but not behind the wheel; I am just sitting back and enjoying the ride. We meander through unfamiliar city neighborhoods, picking up or dropping off other disabled people. I am impressed with how well people manage their properties. I love the city's sounds and the hustle and bustle of life!

> *"Things will be great when you're downtown"*
> *sung by Petula Clark*

Back here: Little voices in the hallways and squeals of laughter outside from the children at daycare delight us. Their playfulness and joy remind us of our grand and great-grandchildren.

We hear the kitchen staff preparing the dining room for another meal.

Sounds I miss and can't go running after, yet! The sound of your voice, your laughter, the music of church bells, a train whistle, cheers at a ball field, the roar of the surf, flagpoles, a lawnmower, a waterfall.

Physical and Occupational Therapies: A Road to Recovery

This facility's care, support, and exercise were never tailored to GBS. How could they have been, given that no one here was an expert in the do's and don'ts of treating this condition?

When I was in so much pain, and the meds wore off way too soon, I was reminded by those witnessing my torment and drama to "just breathe," as though the mere act of doing so would bring fast relief.

One day, after hearing that advice one time too many, I retorted to the nurse, "Do you know how ridiculous you sound?" It felt absurd to be offered this easy remedy for such intense, overwhelming, and overpowering pain. She apologized, and then I apologized to her. Soon afterward, together we tried deliberate, controlled breathing exercises to work through the pain. This did help.

Eventually, the facility beautifully managed my pain from GBS. However, with GBS, priority should also have been given to developing a plan early on to build muscle strength and mobility, as well as a process for assessing progress from the start of my stay.

For months, I was an inert mass, lying in bed, waiting for the meds to dull my pain. My thoughts would go to a dim place, one of having a broken body in need of recovery while also having an active mind, one bent on getting out of long-term care.

"This can't be happening," I begged.

A miracle: One day, a nurse came to ask me if I'd like to be a part of a new exercise program, one designed for residents like me, that would help strengthen muscles and restore some movement.

"Yes, yes, a thousand times, yes!" I responded.

The Site: A Skilled Nursing Facility

The Restorative Program

We tried a little physical therapy a few months into my stay here. However, I contracted COVID and was isolated; once COVID passed, any PT was discontinued, as insurance would not pay for more sessions, having made no progress in mobility!

But then, about four months after arriving at this SNF, this new rehabilitation program began, one designed for bedridden residents and others to get their muscles moving freely and easily again. At the time, I had started to believe I would spend the rest of my days with a highly weakened body but a very active mind; it was not a good place to be.

This new initiative for disabled residents is called The Restorative Program, and it encourages residents to build up their strength and muscles (and nerves) through a series of leg and arm exercises, foot and leg massage, and hand and finger-strengthening exercises. (FYI, Guillain-Barré patients exhibit numbing and tingling sensations in their extremities, pain, and extreme sensitivity when toes and fingers are touched).

The head of the program, Conrad, worked with me every day for a few minutes for months. He worked with me until I could sit up in bed, sit on the side of the bed, and then, using the Hoyer, get into a chair and sit for an hour, which eventually became six hours.

At the same time, the head of PT ordered a pair of straightening boots to wear as often as I could withstand their attempt to hold my legs and feet straight enough to align my feet after they had contracted inward. Suddenly, I was trying to stand up in those boots while holding onto the parallel bars, with help from, Colin, who believed in me and told me I could do it!

Sea Change

After months and months and months of seemingly SLOW progress, the following began to fall into place: little to no muscle/nerve pain; some flexibility in the use of fingers, hands, and arms; generally greater upper body strength and movement; socks tolerated, then shoes; ability to bend the knees and twirl the feet up and down and around; higher leg lifts, and other advances! There became a sense of "being in the real world" once again through rides in the van via stretcher, at first, and then in a wheelchair.

During my first outing, I thought, "So this is my neighborhood, and all these people are my neighbors!"

With my ability to ride in a vehicle came long-awaited visits to my kids' house to see my gorgeous, giggly grandchildren and those adored and adorable dogs. Sitting outside in the middle of the day, smelling the scents of spring, of a new beginning, warmed my heart.

The song "Today" by the great John Denver came to mind, "A million tomorrows shall all pass away, 'ere I forget all the joy that is mine today."

Today brought other close family members and cherished friends (it is always a treat to see them) carrying Tobies Donuts, Subway sandwiches, and bags of goodies to the SNFs patio. What a delight!

The Site: A Skilled Nursing Facility

An important aside: Don't you think a rise from the ashes indicates the kind of care I've received at this facility?

A quick summary of a series of steps toward greater mobility at this facility. In my case, as I said, each small step played out over weeks and months of therapy and included:

- Placing pillows on the bed in an order that would allow me to tolerate pain from any position before needing readjustment.

- Setting a schedule for pills, same pills-same time to dull the pain. The big guns at first included Fentanyl, Oxycodone, and Medical Cannabis.

- Reaching a stage of little or no pain with only the use of Gabapentin, Tylenol, muscle relaxants, and vitamins for comfort.

- Developing a regimen of muscle-building exercises and continuing leg, feet, and toe massage.

- Achieving an upright position and then sitting on the side of the bed to eat.

- Using a sling and Hoyer to move into a wheelchair (kind of a carriage or buggy). So frightening at first!

- Learning to hold a spoon to eat by myself.

- Pushing the buttons on the phone using numb and sore fingers.

- Holding a pen and signing my name on a medical document. Is that my signature now?

- Trying to wash my face, brush my teeth, comb my hair, pluck my eyebrows, and finally put on some lipstick. Oh, joy!
- Applying lotion or spraying on perfume. A luxury!
- Struggling to put on socks and pants.
- Standing up with assistance at the parallel bars.

> Colin, head of Physical Therapy at this facility, and Conrad, head of The Restorative Program, were instrumental in turning things around health-wise during my stay here. Their strategies built a firm foundation for strengthening my physical capabilities while ensuring a healthy mindset, enabling me to begin fighting this limiting condition. The methods were spot-on and carried out with expertise, consistency, and humor. Thanks, guys!
>
> Conrad, you are my main man walking! You are a treasure! Thanks for providing some follow-through at the facility – of all I am learning at Courage Kenny. Our walk-talks you direct so artfully distract me enough to pick up my pace and avoid concentrating on how far it is to the next target landmark! We need to walk more often and for longer periods.

"In the depth of winter, I finally found there was, within me, an invincible summer."
Albert Camus

The Site: A Skilled Nursing Facility

Some of the odds were defied. How many others in long-term care are simply written off with few or no opportunities for even some recovery from their particular maladies?

Moving On: Physical Therapy and Occupational Therapy at Courage Kenny

Having made surprising progress in PT and OT at this facility, and given that insurance had just run out, my family once again contacted Courage Kenny as the most natural next step in my recovery—not only because of their expertise and success in rehabilitating patients but also because of their understanding of GBS.

We first met with Dr. Idiculla, a physical medicine and rehabilitation physician, to assess where things stood with my muscle strength and mobility at this stage. We decided to request entry to CK as an inpatient, as living within the facility would include more frequent opportunities for therapy. Dr. Idiculla said he would make such a recommendation, but the decision was not solely his. After some back and forth with Admissions there, our request for inpatient status was denied.

It was denied because, if approved, I would be coming to them from a Skilled Nursing Facility rather than a hospital, preferably an Allina hospital, under whose auspices CK resides. Rules must always be followed, and they too often involve insurance: who covers what and why.

It was suggested, however, that being an outpatient, one who came to CK a couple of days a week for short (but challenging) sessions would be possible. Sign me up! And that happened almost immediately. And so I transitioned from PT and OT here to CK and their experts, with my promise to give the opportunity everything I had.

CK Recap

Physical Therapy includes getting up in the easy lift, wearing bigger-sized sneakers, being measured for custom-made leg braces, learning to stand in them and pivot while wearing them, walking with them using a regular walker, and practicing walking 30, 60, 250, 300, even 400 feet!

Occupational Therapy involves practicing finger exercises, including playing the piano, using therapy putty, trying out core-strengthening exercises on the mat and using the toilet. A big part of this therapy involves learning to adjust the wheelchair, detach the arm and footrests, and push myself around. I also have had to learn to put on and remove my braces myself. As one's hand and back strength increase, all becomes easier.

I am indebted to my doctor, therapists, and therapy at Courage Kenny!

> Dr. Arun Idiculla is a physical medicine and rehabilitation physician in Minneapolis and is affiliated with Abbott Northwestern Hospital. Dr. Idiculla is highly skilled in assessing patients' symptoms and administering treatments. When he walked through the door for our first meeting, my family and I knew that my life was about to change. We felt assured that help and expertise about GBS were on the way! He is personable and easy to connect with because he listens! He explains things thoroughly and in understandable terms. He is

The Site: A Skilled Nursing Facility

> empathetic; he will go to bat for you, supporting and advocating for you in any way he can.

The Therapists

Courage Kenny's accredited and licensed physical and occupational therapists have given me a new lease on life! For the past six months, I have received their knowledge and expertise in dealing and interacting with patients with neurological conditions and the effects of these conditions on the body's muscles and nerves. Their many strategies, techniques, and apparatuses have helped immensely improve this patient's general fitness and mobility.

So, I move easier and better! I am stronger and more flexible due to their bright, focused, and compassionate work. I've marveled at their willingness as professionals to always get to work, listen to any health updates, keep detailed records of each therapy session, share information with their colleagues, confer about future expectations and plans, and have low-key conversations!

Every disabled person should be given the golden opportunity to go to a Courage Kenny site. Everyone needing physical rehabilitation deserves a chance to work hard, make noticeable progress, and resume some semblance of daily life.

> Courage Kenny's physical therapy therapists, Nathanyal and Kelsie: You made me believe I could walk and devised a plan to ensure that would happen! I am so grateful. You are both experts at what you do.

> Emily: I love our occupational therapy sessions together. They are filled with high expectations, hard work, and great conversations. You are very dear to me.
>
> Sarah: Notice to all! Call Sarah if you feel like you are drowning and there is only a vast and empty sea around you. Oh wait, she's already calling you! A remarkable social worker.
>
> Winkley Ortho: Thank you, Chad, for making my braces. Without them, my legs would be quite useless. With them, I'm beginning to fly!

I am so proud to be a CK patient! Put my photo—braces and all—on a Courage Kenny t-shirt. I'll gladly wear it everywhere and be a "walking" advertisement for this fine institution!

PT and OT Milestones

> *"In the owl's eyes, we see the power of perseverance."*
> *author unknown*

GBS patients must overcome pain, muscle weakness, and fatigue through regular physical and occupational therapies, exercises that build strength and stamina, and appropriate equipment that promotes flexibility and increases mobility.

Here are some of my stellar moments in treatment at the Skilled Nursing Facility and at CK so far that have affected both my physical and emotional health, milestones reached over months

The Site: A Skilled Nursing Facility

of therapy. This progress occurred when I was mainly past the pain of GBS and beyond the fear of "Will I ever walk again?"

- Allowing foot, leg, and toe massages - without squealing - to relax muscles.

- Feeling strong enough to get up by myself and sit on my own on the side of the bed for breakfast. I suddenly could see that infamous "path forward." Things had changed, and more progress would be made.

- Using the scary Hoyer and two aides to lift me into the wheelchair, I would sit for an hour first, then two, then four hours, and more.

- Having the strength to stand up using the parallel bars with support from my PT guys.

- Standing for the first time at CK when someone brought a full-length mirror so I could see my body. I looked like a person! It was an incredible moment.

- Being transported to the doctor's office for an appointment in a wheelchair rather than dead-like on a stretcher!

- Wearing Tortoise and Hare sneakers one size larger (my brother and sister-in-law's shop in Duluth) for the first time in a long time. Cool!

- Walking, albeit unassuredly, with braces custom-made for my advanced contracted legs and feet and a walker.

- Walking with the leg braces and a walker 60 feet, pivoting, and repeating that four times. Walking 300 feet and scoring a touchdown!

Today, I can amble carefully and a bit clumsily over 500 feet nonstop with specially made leg braces and a walker. My therapy will continue for months, and I will walk again unaided! Thanks to God for the miracles of physical therapy!

"How Great Thou Art!" sung by Carrie Underwood

Note: The above highlights the importance of any rehabilitation facility's physical and occupational therapy know-how and offerings.

Site Selection Criteria

And so, with great reluctance, we may consider another place to live besides our home only if we are old, sick, and/or need extra care and support that our families cannot provide. A Skilled Nursing Facility offers an alternative, and long-term care is one of its options.

The challenging journey to find a good place of care and support for Mom, Dad, Gramma, Aunt Jane, yourself, etc., begins with conversations with family about their needs and preferences. This conversation extends to include friends, neighbors, co-workers, and anyone who has ever been down this road and who might offer invaluable insights about which sites to consider and why.

The Site: A Skilled Nursing Facility

Requesting help from a social worker, organizations that work on behalf of the elderly, experienced attorneys who deal with such matters, church elders, or hospital personnel will also increase your knowledge about SNFs and help you make sound, final decisions about any appropriate facility or group of facilities.

These sources can yield several facilities to check out. Visit their websites for their offerings, layout, key people, and general information. A scheduled tour can make each facility more real and present a contrast between those on your list for consideration. It will also give you a good chance to ask questions of facility representatives. (Remember that it is their job to present the rosiest picture).

Be aware that what you learn provides only basic information about each facility. We may easily surmise that "It looks like a good place," "The people seem nice," or "I like their list of resident activities."

Most of us cannot find the time to investigate each facility on our list. Sometimes, we just don't know which questions to ask, as we've probably never done this before. We may not know what will illuminate the essential inner workings of any establishment. Some of these assessments can only be made from a resident's point of view.

Check out the following website for the Minnesota Nursing Home Report Card, which provides information about your choices, including star ratings for resident quality of life, family satisfaction, and inspection results at nhreportcard@dhs.mn.gov. Note: Please do not make any decision based on this information alone!

There are elements of a former, more ordinary, and familiar life found at SNFs among those doing their jobs well. Similarly, there are routines and rituals here - three meals per day, a once-a-week shower, pill and med distribution, and an array of activities to choose to participate in most days. There are rules to abide by, people to interact with (some to merely tolerate), accommodations to evaluate, financial questions to answer, family concerns to address, exercise options, and other well-being suggestions to consider—just like at home!

Undoubtedly, the setting makes it a somewhat different way of life from what we are used to and comfortable with. At a long-term care facility, freedom and choices are limited, but in decent, reputable SNFs like this one, life can be more than tolerable and not too awful—for we are still alive! We are also fortunate if we are attended to by both qualified and certified staff who care to get us well again and/or less disabled.

Additional Pointers for Selecting Your Facility

In selecting a skilled nursing site (which will most likely depend upon availability), be cognizant of many important considerations, including whether or not the site is close to where at least one family member lives. And if the place is near to or easily accessible for friends to visit. Are you exploring some facility that is in a small town or an urban area? Does the neighborhood have a suburban or country vibe to it? How busy is the location you are looking into with traffic? Does the resident-to-be prefer quiet nights or nights filled with the sounds of sirens and motorcycles?

As Neil Diamond sang, *"What a beautiful noise, comin' up from the street, got a beautiful sound, it's got a beautiful beat."*

Which facility and which floor of the facility is available? How are floors and units divided, and for which type of resident, candidates for physical rehabilitation, those needing long-term care, memory care, etc.?

Is the room available a single or a double room? Is there a window in the room assigned? What is there to watch from the window, e.g., wildlife, a neighbor working to perfect a beautiful garden, a bus route, trucks loading and unloading goods? Is the room close to the nurses' station? Is there a visitors' sitting room nearby?

Are the halls clean and free of clutter or equipment? Does the place, as a whole, smell good? Is staff friendly and respectful, and do they interact with residents? Is music playing somewhere, anywhere?

If these considerations seem picky, please know that the prospective resident, whose stay may be extensive, will appreciate your attention to such matters.

What items from home will be suitable for the new place? Consider the size of items and space the room offers, especially the anticipated bureau and closet. Decide what is necessary and proper for daily living that the facility may not provide, and know which selected items from home will give you the most comfort.

Please note: The availability of rooms within certain selected facilities within some geographic regions will strictly limit the number of choices of facilities that can be added to your list. Facilities that are both convenient and accessible.

Making a final decision about the "right place" is a burdensome responsibility and can be daunting. We must use what (little) we've learned to help us select a "home," for that is what it will be for the resident-to-be. The decision is a weighty one, and it should be.

If you plan to dig deep into a prospective facility, here are some questions to consider:

- How does management interact with residents? What channels are available to address residents' rights? Who explains these things to residents and their families?

- What are the qualifications of executive staff? Who's on the Board of Directors? What was the latest year's financial/annual report?

- Who makes the laws and regulations for Skilled Nursing Facilities?

- Who develops the facility's policies? Who is responsible for implementing them? How are they assessed for effectiveness? How effective are they in reflecting residents' needs?

- What is the difference between management and leadership?

Make a clear distinction between leadership and facility management.

A few additional management concerns to think about in making decisions about the "right" facility for your prospective resident:

- Is coffee available to residents and families anytime or only at mealtime? After all, this is Minnesota!
- Does every resident's room have a fan or two to help circulate the air?
- Are snacks given to residents upon request, and may they be at odd hours?
- Is the facility's staff augmented by cheerful volunteers who help with many tasks?
- Who helps residents with hair maintenance and nail care? With shaving? What does reimbursement for these services entail?

Facility Management and Leadership

All Skilled Nursing Facilities have a management team and managers in charge of this and that. All organizations depend upon management to achieve their goals. Management functions include conducting needs assessments, devising an action plan for the organization, making decisions, utilizing resources, recruiting and overseeing personnel, communicating, and assessing effectiveness.

Running a facility may seem far removed from actual caregiving; however, tending to required County and State paperwork and assisting with financial matters and forms necessitated by being a nursing facility is an equally critical form of resident care.

A pervading point of view needs to be addressed. There is a frequent lament that a disconnect (at times, a considerable crevice) exists between the caregivers and management about what those in charge deem necessary for predominant organizational success and what those who work most closely with the clients/customers/patients/residents would prioritize if asked. It manifests itself in a seemingly deliberate choice by some in management positions to ignore the advice, skill, and expertise of those on staff. In these situations, management conveys to all that they know what's best and will make the major decisions, with few requests for "input from staff." This may pertain to setting the direction for the entity, selecting its equipment, training staff, and deciding on in-service strategies.

This facility's management departments include Business Administration, Spiritual Care, Nursing, Admissions, Social Services, Dietetics, Laundry, Medical Records, Recreational and Physical Therapies, Housekeeping, and General Maintenance. House managers meet every morning at 9 AM and hold other meetings as needed.

Leadership, including the Board of Directors and parent company executives, is responsible for leading the charge and fulfilling the organization's mission. It also manages many administrative tasks, hires new staff members, and oversees their work. Leadership must prioritize the safety and care of its residents. Effective and efficient facility management is reflected in its rank within a rating system compared to other facilities in the area or statewide. Satisfied residents and their families further promote it.

You should know the members of the nonprofit facility's Board of Directors and have a snapshot of their backgrounds. You should also know how board members are selected (by nomination?) and their roles and responsibilities, such as helping to fulfill the organization's mission, outreach to the community, fundraising, financial oversight, and knowledge of nonprofit laws and regulations.

Age & Experience: An Owl's Viewpoint

"The person who has lived the most is not the one with the most years, but the one with the richest experience."
Jean-Jacques Rousseau

I beg you to consider the importance of both age AND experience of those put in charge of our Skilled Nursing Facilities. We residents—Owls—can legitimately comment on both, with an emphasis on "experience."

Note: The earned credentials and field experience of those in charge are not being questioned or downplayed.

Age

We may be "old and grey and full of sleep" (William Butler Yeats), yet, the years, the sheer number of years we have lived, have given us insight, intuition, and perspective in our ability to assess situations and make correct calls about them. We are oftentimes—surprisingly quick—to comprehend circumstances and conditions with clarity and comprehension. We are even better at sizing-up individuals, as it relates to their job competence and skill.

Experience

What is there to be said about having "experience" that can translate into wisdom?

> *"You cannot create experience. You must undergo it."*
> *Albert Camus*

Wisdom comes only through experience, particularly those experiences that test us, our strength, resiliency, and judgment.

The more years we have, the more time we are given to figure out how to best cope with the unexpected—the most challenging, difficult, and overwhelming situations that require us to lean into our experience and accumulated knowledge to solve persistent problems. The more experience we gain, the better we become at using what we know.

Wisdom

Acquiring knowledge takes a long time. No one I know in their twenties or even early thirties has amassed a depth of knowledge in their respective careers (Olympians aside) about most anything; they are just beginning to discover what works and what won't.

Some say that the peak years of one's career are when individuals are in their late 40's or early 50's. Wisdom tells us that our Skilled Nursing Facilities need those who are at the top of their professional lives to "keep a course, maneuver correctly, and steer the ship." Lives are at stake here!

Mentors

Hanging out with those who are more experienced—who have learned over time and are skilled at making decisions and planning actions, especially those affecting the lives of the very old, very sick, and disabled in Skilled Nursing Facilities—is a must for those new to being at the helm.

Usually, those seeking optimal career experience are paired with mentors who are available and eager to share what they have learned—perhaps the hard way. Mentoring those new to any job is critical to their success, confidence, and credibility.

Seeking out the best to imitate, learn from, and listen to—those with more miles and experience—demonstrates maturity and reassures top management that they have the role models and support needed to learn, grow, and succeed. It also ensures they can apply the knowledge they are constantly gaining.

Please consult us Owls about anything; we just might be able to contribute to the dialogue.

Families

What is it about those in charge of a facility that inspires residents to have confidence in them—their knowledge, intuition, judgment calls, plans, and coordination, as well as their mentors, team, and sincere desire to improve the lives of those they serve? The bottom line: What experience qualifies them to run the show?

3

The Residents:
The Centerpiece of Any Facility

Who Are We?

I am sitting working at the (only) desk available for paperwork, which is in an alcove that precedes yet another hallway with a set of resident rooms. I hear some crying, and recognize ——'s voice, talking to her friend on the phone. She says, "I don't have anyone to talk to" (she lives in a single room) - in such a pathetic, reedy high-pitched voice, I wanted to cry along with her. This was followed by an even louder, stronger, and rousing lament, one filled with distress and defiance: "I AM A PERSON!!"

That is who we are.

We are lone birds in a tree (in an SNF) - each of us is prominent, proud, courageous, and resilient. At rest on a twig before we fly once again.

We are in the last season of life, the winter, and in the stage of life reserved for, and dubbed, the "elderly." These are among the most important years, because they are the final, concluding ones.

Like the birds, we sit, perched against a vast, solitary, graying sky, with a view that affords us a sweeping, unobstructed, undeniable panorama of our life's journey.

And so, we reflect from on high, looking in all directions: back, down, and forward. We've got the "back" and the "down" mastered! The future, we know beyond a doubt, holds so much yet to do, to see, to feel, to learn, and to teach. And there's even room for a bit of flight of fantasy—running, dancing, or even flying!

Look at us! Look again! Once more!

If you do, you will see beyond a first glance that spotlights our age, race, sick and sagging bodies, wrinkles, posture, too-long or too-short hair, outdated clothes, inability to walk or walk easily, clumsiness, or rusty table manners. You will no longer see just a disabled body or a sad face; physical appearance will be of secondary importance. You will see each of us, each bird, separate from the others and as a unique and special someone.

Make the time! Take the time! Turn that first impression around! You will be in for a pleasant surprise! We can still be helpful and valuable to you as you are to us.

"In the eye of an owl, we find the depth of wisdom."
author unknown

We will gladly share what we birds have learned: the importance of respect for others, responsibility, self-control, patience, and kindness; how to slog through life's mud and maintain your dignity; how to solve life's many complicated problems. And more! We can make you laugh! We can listen to, pray, and sing along with you.

If you let us.

All People

As a matter of expediency, we group people—label them—and find a category within which they tend to fall, e.g., women (all women), coworkers, relatives, neighbors, teens, foodies, artists, athletes, and churchgoers—so that we can more easily describe or explain them or sometimes dismiss them as though that is who they are or only are!

Vast swaths of people include individuals with similarities that make "grouping" possible. And, with closer scrutiny, it may point out stark differences between and among individuals within each group. Too often, we use a broad stroke to describe a particular mass of people (often in harmful ways) by avoiding or omitting any detailed information that would separate individuals within each group in various ways, especially positively.

For example, it's just easier to slap a label on "those past sixty," which itself is a fact, but one that may conjure up some imprecise, inaccurate, or false description as "less than" and omit other critical information about them, i.e., their lives, livelihoods, values, likes and dislikes, their experience, their opinions.

Designating individuals in general terms or by a particular name (team, social group, organization, or club) or illness only makes it easier and more probable to misunderstand, misperceive, and misinterpret them in significant ways within the group.

The Aging and Aged

We all age chronologically, but people age in different ways. Aging affects people's bodies and minds in various ways. Some of those who are sorted as "elderly" and "aged" still "work," travel the world, play pickleball, serve on committees or volunteer (in a host of ways), canoe, paint on canvas, photograph birds and wildlife, faithfully attend exercise classes, sing in choirs, and tend to grandchildren.

They move: no flies on them!

Some of these elderly people have not dealt with a significant illness. Others in this grouping have had health concerns already, have sufficiently recovered, and yet may face further apparent physical and/or mental decline in the future. The degree to which individuals experience such decline varies, but it will eventually limit one's options and possible contributions to life.

With such decline comes the care and support necessary to sustain life. The amount and type of care these elderly individuals require depends on their physical and mental (and emotional) health and well-being. Those who need the most care and support, usually for a longer time, are often housed in Skilled Nursing Facilities in long-term care.

It sounds like the most dire, end-of-the-road situation!

It can be, but it is not a sure thing! Despite one's physicality or mental acumen deterioration, the spirit remains. And, because it is so, together with exceptional nursing and management care and support, a means of rallying exists and is a powerful force for change - towards better and improved health, in general, once again. DO NOT EVER DISCOUNT THESE EXCEPTIONAL SURVIVORS!

The Residents of This SNF

Not only do we find ourselves in a new place, we are sick, and some of us are disabled or both. We may have been moved suddenly and find ourselves in a strange new world. We feel homesick; nothing is familiar.

"The ache for home lives in all of us." Maya Angelou

It takes getting used to this loss of control in our lives and activities. We think of it as accepting new activities and challenges, those relating to our health and well-being, rather than our former fun and adventurous activities over which we had some control.

We mourn our significant loss, the loss of what was, of life as we knew it. We yearn for the times we spent with family and as a family.

"In life, you have to make the most of any situation."
John Daly

A reminder to each of us in the care of a Skilled Nursing Facility, *"You are braver than you believe, stronger than you seem, and smarter than you think."* A.A. Milne

Who Were We?

Residents here at this facility fall into one of two categories: short-term, transitional care, or long-term care, which includes memory care.

Residents are from many walks of life and include a former taxicab driver, an IT and computer expert, a sculptor, the first woman veterinarian at the University of Minnesota, a renowned geneticist, a school teacher, a composer, a TSA agent, an Ohio GM executive, an automotive specialist, a juvenile court service supervisor, former chaplains, homemakers, a college professor, nurse's aides, and farmers.

Our Lives in Themes

Music

The years of romantic love seem to fly by and last but a second. Time spent in a long-term care facility can drag as we linger.

Mark Twain said, "Humor is the great thing, the saving thing after all." I say that honor goes to MUSIC.

Music recalls a particular time, a happening, a place, or a person. It stirs our emotions, eliciting longing, contentment, and nostalgia for our past.

This phenomenon is perfectly captured in Trisha Yearwood's rendition of Hugh Prestwood's "The Song Remembers When."

"...I heard that old familiar music start.
It was like a lighted match

The Residents: The Centerpiece of Any Facility

Had been tossed into my soul..."

When I was a young girl and then an emotional teen, I used the piano to express my true feelings of anticipation, happiness, anger, sadness, disappointment, or fear. While playing, I was not analyzing which emotion I was playing; the songs I chose simply served my mood best at the time. As a wife, mother, and grandmother, music made (makes) fussing and worrying easier!

"Music was my refuge." Maya Angelou

As older adults, listening to music can make us feel less alone and help us recall wonderful memories. Older people have incredible long-term memories that easily retrieve thoughts of good times and laughter from long ago. Our preferred music genre, especially, affects our minds and bodies in good ways, and fills our hearts.

Music reminds us to 'be of good cheer'—to have hope, not get discouraged, not lose faith, and (try to) live a life of joy' (The Church of Latter-day Saints). How important is that mindset, especially at our age!

When we are upset or anxious, music can help us relax and encourage us to step back from current health concerns; it soothes us in soft ways. Music helps us to "let go" happily, even briefly, of all that is too weighty.

A Most Happy Day

My occupational therapist, Emily, is a violinist. One day, when I arrived at CK, Emily said, "Let's go and find a piano." After two years without my Kawai, I welcomed her suggestion.

She pointed to a book of piano classics, "Play something," she instructed.

I chose "Fur Elise," a favorite of mine. And so, with my body in position, and despite my numb and tingling fingers, I played, with clinkers apparent and with the hesitancy of one's first recital. I didn't play well, but I played. Apologies to Herr Beethoven! And love to my Emily for knowing how important that gesture of hope was to me!

Back at the facility, Mary Ann, the Associate Pastor here, and others from management have arranged for me to play the Chapel's grand piano. They move the piano in place each time I play so I can get my feet positioned without braces to use the pedals. My fingers have loosened up, and there has been some noticeable improvement in my playing to the point where there is now a sound of music! Practice makes perfect? We'll see!

Activities

Thanks to staff members Alyssa, Sarah, Nick, and Grace, as well as resident volunteers who diligently plan and carry out a full array of activity options for all interested residents each month. Options have included learning about life in other countries; prayer services and Bible study; music trivia; Karaoke; Spanish classes; balloon volleyball; bowling or Bocce Ball; card games;

therapy dog visits; Jeopardy; art projects such as drawing, painting, and ceramics. And BINGO!

With such a long list, surely one can find at least two activities of interest to attend. These activities provide a nice opportunity to mingle with other residents. Bringing in guest speakers or performers elevates our spirits!

Activities occur throughout the facility, mainly in the Chapel or one of the dining rooms. We can choose to help plan them, watch them, participate in, or be entertained by them.

There are always those from the Activities staff who come to remind each of us about a forthcoming activity. They encourage our attendance but are not pushy! Bill is our "wheelchair chauffeur," getting us easily from place to place.

The Elderly and God

At our age, we all look for something to hold on to (just in case?). Most residents are people of faith who may move even closer to God as they age. Most feel that someone is in charge of the world, someone who knows what He is doing! Because of this belief, residents may feel less fearful and more trusting.

You can hear from residents that "God is good!" Or, "Praise be to God!" Or, "God's got it!" (Don't worry!).

Members of their respective churches visit some of the residents. These fellow churchgoers bring laughter and goodwill and say prayers aloud for the person they've come to see—for better health and peace.

Religion

Residents of SNFs represent many ethnicities, e.g., White, African American, Asian, Hispanic, Latino, Native American.

Most facilities have representatives of different religions, such as Christianity, Islam, Judaism, Hinduism, and Buddhism. Nonbelievers, the irreligious, and those unsure of their position on the issue, may also be members of a facility's community.

There may be specific differences in religious practices. Still, most residents share a common belief in a supreme being—a creator who is all-knowing (a justifiable know-it-all!) and all-powerful, having made us and the universe. There is a strong sense of assurance that this being will save us, transform us (and our circumstances), empower us, and forgive our transgressions. We turn to Him in search of comfort, companionship, and acceptance of who we are now.

Like most readers, I've walked through many fires in my lifetime. I know I've never walked through them alone.

Talking with God

A prayer is something to grasp onto, hold tightly to, and revel in - its promised power.

It's a very good thing to know that you can instantly converse with the All-powerful, who is always there for you and, when you talk, will listen.

In communicating with God, I sometimes recite prayers I've said all my life – knowing them each so well, I often fail to pay attention to each word, like playing a song you've played repeatedly on the piano and forgetting to make each note count.

When I need help working through a concern or problem, when I feel hopeful, forgiving, or grateful, or when I need to ask for something I desperately need or want, I aim for a less formal but longer, more thoughtful, and more impassioned talk with God (and with some who reside with Him).

Both ways of conversing bring comfort, strength, and even healing.

> *Prayer works its magic by reducing fear—especially the fear of change, which is so prevalent at this stage of our lives.*

There is something unique about prayer: it can happen whenever we choose and for as long as we want. In this, we wield such unusual control!

Emotions: What Are We Feeling?

Loneliness and Aloneness

We at the facility are fully aware that, at first glance, we are seen as a group of weakened older folks in need. This is a fact! That observation aside, however, we consider ourselves distinct individuals with inner strengths, such as patience and adaptability, that go beyond the obvious.

As individuals, as human beings, though ill or infirm, we continue to experience human emotions like happiness, gratitude, inspiration, sadness, anger, pride, fear, disappointment, or shame.

This brings us to loneliness, another noteworthy emotion, and to feeling alone.

No one has a corner on loneliness, aloneness, or on feeling lonely. Loneliness is akin to feeling happy or sad; try telling someone happy or sad not to be so! Such feelings are natural and universal. They occur regardless of how close we are to our spouse, children, other family members, and friends (even best friends).

Several years ago, I had a friend, Amy, who had a friend, Mike, who planned to move across the country and sell some of his possessions. Alongside those for purchase were a few marked "not for sale." Of course, I was most interested in those items, especially the artwork!

In the not-for-sale section, on a far wall, I spied a medium-sized painting of a relatively small blackbird sitting in a barren tree. There was nothing but the bird and the tree in the picture. The starkness of a lone bird against a sky of grey and pale yellows drew me like no other. I felt an immediate affinity to it! Had I been the artist, it would have been a self-portrait!

My interpretation of the painting was not one of feeling sorrow for the bird's aloneness or of the possibility that fellow birds rejected or abandoned it. It was not of it being cruelly left behind or adrift. It did not conjure up any pity. The painting, instead, spoke to me of strength and grace, courage, dignity, acceptance, and peace found despite its current state, as depicted. It was not lonely, as much as it was alone.

Mike did not want to part with it! I begged, and he relented. The painting has stayed with me and has been prominently displayed for decades. Though now in storage, I still feel its message, influence, and power—maybe especially now, ***as the bird is, to me, every resident of this facility!***

There are times in all our lives, of course, when we have felt the squeeze in our gut, the ache of "being in this," whatever "this" is, by ourselves - and that ultimately, each of us must see "this thing" through, alone. (Even though there may be loving and supportive people around us).

As we age, we certainly feel alone or lonely as we lose some of our identity: our working lives, familiar surroundings, and regular activity schedules. We simply, unapologetically, and profoundly miss these extremely important things! This can make us teeter but not fall.

At times, we must follow through with what others expect of us or with commitments we've made: to cross the finish line, to give a speech, to fulfill a promise made, to give birth! At such times, each of us stands alone. We must find within ourselves the faith, courage, and strength to do it and go it alone.

One such time, for any of us residents, may be now.

Anger

Humans experience a range of emotions; we emote in different ways and to varying degrees.

Any emotion we feel at a particular time can be so apparent to others that they just have to look at our expressions. For example, a happy face, with a broad smile and flashing eyes, is instantly noticeable, heartwarming, and reflective of great joy.

Anger, too, is unmistakable, evidenced by a frown, furrowed brow, scowl, or glare. It is not a pretty look.

Anger says, "Stop it!" "Knock it off!" "Get lost!" "Take a hike!" Anger shouts, "What do you mean?" Or, "How dare you!" A simple "Damn it!" speaks volumes!

No one would describe the residents at this facility as angry. But, of course, as individuals and humans, we all get angry, occasionally. The feeling is quite common, instinctive, and rather ordinary.

While I have witnessed "resident anger" here, it manifests as annoyance, displeasure, or disappointment with something or someone. It has never remotely come close to being a fit of rage or a temper tantrum, and it is very seldom even a rant or a rave.

Resident-observed displays of anger here have been infrequent, restrained, and/or short-lived. In our golden years, we can better consider our actions before we strike out at anything that has perturbed us or anyone we find disagreeable or too controlling.

However, it can suddenly burst forth as if a dam has broken! The release of such can be a healthy thing! Venting and cursing loudly (poppin' the cork!) can relieve stress and clear the air. "It built up and just needed to come out!" We project our anger through our words, not through physical altercations.

The Residents: The Centerpiece of Any Facility

When we strike out at someone or about anything, the root cause may have us festering about a matter far more important than what we've just railed at or against. For residents, the basis for our anger (I think) originates (and simmers) because most of us: 1) have contracted a severe, debilitating disease, which we may or may not be familiar with or understand; and 2) (we) have been sent to an SNF for care, and have had to leave our beloved home.

Yes, we are angry about that! No apologies! Both have changed our way of life in monumental ways.

Here are some examples of what gets us riled up to the point of sounding off, and we just have to say something!

> A resident: "I woke up to find a member of staff rifling through my closet looking for a particular pair of jeans- without my permission. That really ticked me off!" (What's mine is yours?)
>
> Another: "I waited an hour and a half after pressing the call light to be taken to the bathroom and changed." Ridiculous!
>
> A resident about another resident: "I can't listen to her yell, 'Come on, Supper,' or 'Professor!' one more time!" My limit is 30 times within a two-hour timeframe.
>
> An aide took supplies from my drawer after he thought I was asleep. I don't mind sharing critical supplies with other residents, but why are we in short supply so often?
>
> Resident: "What's with the food? It's tasteless, predictable, and inconsistent with my dietary preferences."
>
> Residents: Financial matters between residents and management should be discussed behind closed doors, not in

> resident rooms when a roommate is present or at the facility's front desk!
>
> Resident: "Over the past several months, I've met with social workers and a couple outside the facility regarding a possible move. When I see them, I ask if a place has been found for me in Assisted Living. (I signed some paperwork for one facility.) How much longer will I have to wait to get some straight answers? I've been very patient until now." (So frustrating, as she may no longer require long-term care)
>
> Another: "For months, I've been promised a telephone. Where is it? I need a phone to call my lawyer, doctor's office, and friends living in other states."
>
> Resident to resident: "Didn't you say your doctor ordered some physical therapy for you? When do you start?" "I haven't heard a thing." No response is deadly to a resident. This roadblock prevents residents from moving forward and progressing, leaving them "treading water."
>
> Resident: "When is the Resident Doctor's next visit? I've been waiting for weeks to see him! Am I on his list of residents to see? No one seems to know."

Are we irked? Confused by a need for more responses to our questions and needs? Mad at the fact that it wouldn't take much to rectify these situations. You bet!

How we vent our anger at others is key. It takes a lot of energy to be angry with someone or about anything. The energy expended in this way can best be used to remain calm (inside and out), keeping blood pressure and heart rates low, and hormone levels in check.

We must also consider the feelings of those we target and whether our anger is fully displayed for others who might not choose to witness it. Going to the source of our anger, in confidence, or to the one who can rectify the bothersome situation might be the best course of action. If not, the toll it takes on the one displaying anger is high: shame, regret, misery, or isolation—for having expressed oneself in this manner.

We are not angry people by nature; we only get angry sometimes!

Hope

So, most of us are people of faith. We believe; we pray. Then, something tough and challenging happens to us. It rocks us, our world. It steps all over everything. And we are down for the count.

Seemingly, out of nowhere, we put up some kind of fight, if only a weak one. Consciously or unconsciously, we resist the difficulty, and we fight back. We toughen up. And feel a sense of power. That power is HOPE. What a gift! It's a breakthrough, a way out, a means to move beyond what is difficult and seemingly insurmountable. It is the sense of something more substantial, mightier, of what can be better.

Hope is a wonderful sense of joy. It is peculiar and can take many forms. What triggers or inspires hope in the residents?

A change of seasons as one season passes, and a new season replaces it with its own impossible uniqueness. As aging adults, we have experienced many seasons and now face a limited number of seasons to come. Hope gives us the courage to accept this reality and to make the most of each season given.

Hope is a new friend.

Hope is a talk with a fellow disabled resident who informs us that he has filed admissions papers for a slot at Courage Kenny, a positive, try-hard-and-succeed goal for his future.

Hope is an acceptable blood sugar level and/or blood pressure reading.

Hope is one big hug!! "That's not a hug! This is a hug!" Ahh!

Hope is a look at one's grandchildren.

Hope is a mighty thing. It can surface when we are simply tired of feeling defeated.

Hope is the passing of a fellow resident, friend, family member (or beloved pet), one we know goes before us to prepare us for when it is our turn.

Walking a few steps, then a few more, and down this new hallway. Hope is progress.

Hope has hall doors wide open and requires no masks.

Hope is finding anything that seems "lost," especially ourselves.

Hope is anticipation. It's a chance to see that same resident friend at mealtime, sitting at the table, waiting to chat.

It is making plans to go home or watching a resident leave the facility for a new "home."

The Residents: The Centerpiece of Any Facility

Hope is shower day! That first cup of coffee! A new love!

It is flower buds and rose petals opening one by one.

Hope is the following, most exciting, three months before Christmas!

Hope is a song! Your smiling face! Your arms, open wide!

Hope makes us believe that something better will happen soon or in the long run. It foretells positive change, a new opportunity, and a forwardness to what might happen, which is emphatically possible.

Faith

The years help erase doubt, and we mightily trust instead. But some questions remain, and we require answers.

Within the vastness of the universe, how big can God's heaven be? Is it so expansive that it spans the length and breadth of the entire cosmos?

Where does God put everyone up there? How does He make room for everyone – the Old Guard and the Newbies alike? Do we need to reconsider the concept of 'space' as limitless, boundless, and unending? Can we even fathom it? How many football fields is that?

When we die and stand waiting at the Pearly Gates besides St. Peter, who will our promised greeters be? A spouse, Mom and Dad, Max, a child, brothers and sisters, good friends or teachers, beloved pups? Those we miss who have gone before us, for sure.

Those whose passing we tolerate but have never fully accepted. We grieve for them, still.

Will there be a crowd or slim line of those who wait to welcome us, who want nothing more than to reunite with us? Or will there be one or two designees who prepared for our arrival? (Perhaps they were in the know as to date and time.)

Will we recognize those we see? What if they are changed in some way? What will they wear—a piece we've seen many times before? Will we immediately sense their familiarity, their love? Will we need to catch up with them on events or happenings? Or is there no need to, as their bird's eye view has seen it all?

Will we see only rows of souls, the spirits of our loved ones, who step out of line to extend their greeting? Who will be the first to do so? Will they radiate joy and happiness? Will they instantly embrace us, saying, "We've waited so long to see you again; what took you so long?"

Will we be instantly reunited with them, officially admitted into heaven, and wholeheartedly immersed in them?

Will we see the face of God?

Will we feel an unquestionable, unequivocal sense of peace? Will its beauty awaken us, our senses?

We believe that all will fall gracefully into place, and there will be room enough for each of us at God's table and in God's heaven.

Issues

Setting Things Right

Residents have a strong need to set things right. We want to ensure our loved ones think about important things should we one day not be around to remind them. We need those we care about to know they are still in our thoughts, even after a long hiatus. We need some of them to know that we regret some of our actions. We, who are being cared for, need our loved ones to know we still care for and support them in some way, even now.

Tying Up Loose Ends

When we reach a certain age, we assess what we've done and left undone. We strive to get things in order, be that our houses, finances, or final wishes.

When we are stuck in a situation or in some place, things that didn't get said or done may more likely bother us; we tend to dwell on them, as we feel these important things require our attention or at least some answers. For example:

One resident is trying to find out what happened to his stepdaughter, who disappeared while suffering from an addiction.

Another's wish is to carry on her work with young minority kids. Not done yet!

One wants to know what happened to a piece of property he prized and who now owns it.

Another asks, "Where is my car?"

I need to call my friend to apologize to her for abandoning our friendship. How cruel was I?

Will my daughter remember to remove the lint from the dryer filter each time the dryer is used? Will she and her husband remember to check the radon gas levels in the house? Will they have the latest innovative fire extinguisher on hand?

Another resident wants to make peace with his son. At this point, he thinks the fight with him was about some inconsequential matter.

Is there still time to contact a former boss who always treated me with respect? Will he even remember me? I need to thank him.

I want my friend, Arnetta, to know how fondly I remember our work with teachers and how much I learned from her.

> *"I never made promises lightly, and there have been some that I've broken."*
> *"Fields of Gold" sung by Eva Cassidy*

What Matters

It's the little things that matter! (Or so it says under my high school yearbook picture). Now, once again, I find that the little things—this time those basic yet somehow critical things—seen and heard at a nursing facility can make or break a day! Residents agree and share:

The Residents: The Centerpiece of Any Facility

"My hands don't hurt at all today."
"Pizza for lunch?!"
"The sun is shining so brightly."
"She's in a great mood today!"
"The grass is so green across the street."
"My brothers and sisters-in-law are coming to visit me next Friday!"
"I was talking to a new friend in the lunchroom."
"Mary gave me her blanket."
"Linda found my shirt in the laundry room!"
"My daughter brought me a lipstick to wear!"
"I'm reading this great mystery!"
"The rose bush—so spectacular—across the street reminds me of my mother's garden."
"My red capris!" Found!
"Cherry pie for dessert!"
"I'm wearing earrings again!"

Besides strides made health-wise, the little things make our hearts lighter and our minds clearer. I found my old, tattered, and comfy-cozy, navy-blue sweatshirt hanging in the closet. It says "Georgetown Hoyas" on it. (No, that was not my school.) Like an old shoe, it is! We feel blessed by these small things.

> *"A morning glory at my window satisfies me more than the metaphysics of books."*
> *Walt Whitman*

Waiting

Throughout our lives, we are active as human beings. We are on the move, mostly doing things of consequence, things to revel in and maybe, over time, to regret.

Yet, it seems that we also spend so much time WAITING for something of necessity to happen. For example, we wait to be fed, get older (I want to be 10!), learn to drive, graduate, work, receive a paycheck (wow!), and make our own decisions. We wait for church to begin, in line at the grocery store, or to get the car repaired. We wait to watch a favorite TV show, for a concert to start, or for traffic to unjam. We wait for seasons to pass, our kids to mature, and for flowers to bloom.

We wait patiently for that special someone we will cherish.

We wait—often for a long time–to be acknowledged and appreciated, valued and accepted, to become successful, and always to be loved.

This phenomenon is exacerbated in a Skilled Nursing Facility, where it's all about "the wait." We cannot move things along as much as we'd like, and we must rely on others to choose when they can fulfill our many requests.

Within these walls, the wait is often over small things; however, sometimes, it is about things that could not be more critical, i.e., a fall. The waiting then carries a more pronounced sense of urgency and even a sense of wonderment. For sure, we can grow impatient!

The Residents: The Centerpiece of Any Facility

We await doctors' appointments for information, test results, or a follow-up course of action. We hardly wait to hear, "It's nothing to worry about. See you in three to four months."

We wait for pill time—or exercise time. We wait for the shower room to become vacant, for a shift to change, and for a ready staff to be brought on. We wait for someone to cheerily answer the call light, and for an able-bodied person to move our bodies from place to place, usually from the bed to the wheelchair and back again—going nowhere fast!

We wait daily for a (good) meal, a tray to be picked up, an extra cup of coffee, or more sugar or salt packets (small ones!). We also wait for a scheduled activity: hymn singing, BINGO, an entertainer, Bible study, another puzzle book, or new batteries for the television remote.

We wait for the darkness and quiet of the evening to watch the stars and airplanes flying across the night sky.

We wait for a definite show of progress in our health and well-being, duly noted by all. *Perhaps all is not over yet!*

We wait for a stimulating, intelligent conversation (please!!) or one that helps retrieve a fond memory in time. We say something funny and wait for your laughter.

We wait for and delight in any semblance of normalcy.

Family and friends, we wait to see you, receive and offer you a hug, and feel the warmth and love in your closeness. We wait for you to make it all better, if only for a while.

"Privacy"

Privacy: herein, a fundamental human right, commonly referred to as freedom from observation.

Try to find some! It is hard to have a private conversation or telephone call in this facility for anyone with a disability. There are few places to scurry to quickly that might afford some privacy, but it is even more challenging for someone in a wheelchair. (And everyone can see the elephant in the room!).

What do you do when your family calls with a concern, your bank calls with a question, or a friend's words are meant only for your ears? What should you do when staff or management make unexpected, unannounced visits to air one of their worries that needs immediate attention? Dare to voice a complaint out loud, one meant only for a couple of people at the lunch table, and the words echo across the room.

As in any relatively small facility (or small town), news travels fast, and people will voice their opinions about what they have heard. It is not, however, dwelt upon, and sometimes it is even quickly forgotten here.

There is some privacy within residents' rooms. Still, the raggedy curtains that divide rooms into halves make any conversations that attempt to be hush-hush or ordinary heard by all. On the positive side, curtains can make you think you have your own little space. It feels enclosed but not closed off, private but not too private, especially if your room has a window to the outside world.

But, if you are relatively tidy and keep your side of the room in order, and your roommate needs to do the same with her side, the room seems lopsided! And you may think, *I want to go home!*

Privacy is challenging when living within agreed-upon limits with a roommate you would not necessarily have chosen. It means setting the volume of the TV so as not to disturb somebody sleeping across the curtain, playing music that will be accepted, and spraying the right type and amount of room freshener.

Privacy has a great deal to do with respect for the very private, individual preferences of one's roommate. It means not having any objection to the TV being on all night or acting like the room is a library because your roommate sleeps a lot during the day, and you must be so respectfully quiet. It may mean saying nothing when the window is open all night.

In the dead of night, I think about my father, so tired after a day of work and baseball, in a deep sleep and snoring away; all was well. It is not the same when my roommate snores, though it is a much quieter version of his snoring.

The Good

Sometimes, the walls come down, and there is little need for privacy, and it feels right to share a space. It feels good to be together to share stories about incredible friends, professional successes, or the lives and doings of precious grandchildren; stories about better-forgotten times at school, bad bosses, or lost friends. Or, to share our next big move once we get out of here!

Privacy is about having your very own space, if only at times! But there is nowhere to run! Unless you have a private room, there is no private space except in one's mind. (So, hold tight to those private thoughts, to your privacy, until they just have to become butterflies!)

It must be said—with emphasis—that the nursing staff most often insists upon some amount of resident privacy while tending to delicate matters. The shades are drawn, and all curtains closed; resident confidences and secrets are not shared, and little gossip is spread.

Their professionalism is to be commended. They respect the confidentiality of information about residents' health and any restrictions on sharing health records and reports. Sensitive medical and health matters are kept close here per HIPAA demands (The Health Insurance Portability and Accountability Act of 1996. One of its five parts deals with patient privacy.)

Talk about Privacy: The Use of a Commode

Oooh! They've moved a commode into my room, another sign of my step-by-step progress! Through the therapy offered at CK, with the help of my new leg braces (ouch!), and after weeks of trial and error, I can stand, awkwardly steer my walker, take a few heavy-laden steps, pivot around, and gently sit.

So here I am, NOT sitting on the commode but looking at it, in my 1/2-room, a room that sometimes feels like Grand Central! Usually, visitors are welcomed, with staff dispensing meds, taking blood pressure measurements, stopping to chat, arranging exercise times, or checking to see if we need anything.

So, here the commode sits, and here I sit in my wheelchair, avoiding that thing in my room, with a firm resolve not to humiliate myself further while guaranteeing that my friends and family will visit with me only in the sitting room down the hall!

Location, Location, Location

Why would I take joy in sitting in the open on a commode? At such a time, like anyone else, I want seclusion and solitude beyond that offered by the room's dividing curtain. Refit me with a smaller wheelchair that can easily roll to the bathroom toilet. Something that would allow me to use the handrails to stand and pivot, then sit behind a closed door. There would be some dignity in that; add a good book or magazine to read, and I can feel normal. No interruptions, please!

Changing Diapers

Like with babies – your loved and lovable ones – it must be done! Kudos to those who think nothing of doing so for near-strangers, while maintaining a bit of privacy.

Sociableness

Over the first many months of my stay, I spent time only in my room, so I didn't meet many of the residents. I slept and ate in my room, and because my roommates were ambulatory, I spent most of my days alone.

Now that I can get around in my wheelchair, I have come to know a few of the residents reasonably well. These include Gene, Brad, Al, Jaddie, LaVonne, and Cynthia. We socialize: no need for privacy. Since we are all in the same boat, I feel an affinity to each of them, especially those with the frailest bodies. I wonder how these residents, ravaged by sickness, can be so strong in spirit! Their will to live supersedes any obstacle put in their way.

I admire the three men on our floor who let nothing deter them from their daily walks along the halls with their walkers, sometimes three or more times a day.

Dreams and Dreaming

Because we all sleep, we all dream. Dreams and dreaming are natural phenomena occurring at all stages throughout our lives. Dreams contribute to our mental, emotional, and physical health and well-being. They help us process and/or replay life events, reassess concerns or problems (some of which we've beaten to death when awake), help us understand our emotions, and aid in self-reflection. We don't always remember what or who we dream about.

Here are some dreams residents at this facility remembered:

> Resident: "In my dreams, I am very present. If the wind is blowing, I feel the wind; if it's raining, I feel the rain. It is all so real to me. When I awake, I wonder where I am."
>
> This was from a never-married resident who wished to be: 'I dreamed I was getting married, and on my way to the altar, I didn't stop. I just kept walking toward a bright light, toward

God. So, I wondered, 'God, what are you showing me?' I figured He showed me that I made the right decision to keep walking!' Not now, not this man.

One resident had a dream about the legendary singer Prince. If you remember, Prince respectfully declined to sing on the acclaimed recording of "We Are the World," which was made to raise money for the famine in Africa in 1985. In her dream, upon rethinking his decision, Prince returned to life to do just that, adding his voice to the now notable and influential group of singers. The resident awoke both awestruck and delighted!

In my dreams, I walk; I am never disabled, and simply, normal. No braces, man!

That of a 90-year-old resident: "My dream became a nightmare. I cut loose from here and headed alone to the airport or train station. I was so scared and confused." He seemed so vulnerable.

Many residents' dreams are about their mothers, fathers, and spouses. Dreams allow for a view of the past, which may still be longed for, and a recalling of moments of the most intense, complicated, and ingrained relationships. "Mama, is that you sitting on my bed? You're wearing your plaid dress."

My favorite dream was a lofty one of infinite joy and would be entitled "A Walk with God" (Himself!). In my dream, God and I stroll, hand-in-hand, down a quiet country road! Just the two of us. In the dream, I feel so small but safe. Was it a vision of the future?!

> Resident: "Last night, I dreamed about my dad. I dream about my mom all the time, but not my dad. He didn't have anything to say to me. He was just sitting in the chair." She said her father never really wanted to talk with his children while he was alive.
>
> Another resident: "I had a dream last night that my "not-religious" dad went to heaven. He stood at the gate, watching my mother and sister laughing and having a good time on the inside."
>
> My husband lived to be almost 80. He constantly dreamed of flying, which gave him a high and expansive view of places, people, and their environments. He was a geography professor for many years, and his thirst to see and know about everything was insatiable. He was so powerful, magical, and free!

One thing is for sure: our "nursing home" dreams reflect and encapsulate some of our past selves across a lifetime and our hopes for the future.

We should study the meaning of dreams more and the types of dreams the elderly experience. We might learn more about our residents from their dreams, get a glimpse into the inner workings of the aging mind, and gain more knowledge about the effects of certain prescribed meds on dreams and the like. We might be able to help people better reflect upon and accept the things they cannot seem to forget, or things they cannot quickly overcome, things that manifest themselves in dreams.

Besides, "I had this amazing dream last night" is a great conversation starter at the breakfast table!

Mental Health and the Aged

"Mental health encompasses emotional, psychological, and social well-being. It influences how we think, feel, and act, as well as how we manage stress, connect with others, and make healthy decisions"(Centers for Disease Control and Prevention).

According to the American Psychological Association (APA), mental health is "a state of mind characterized by emotional well-being, good behavioral adjustment, relative freedom from anxiety and disabling symptoms, and a capacity to establish constructive relationships and cope with the ordinary demands and stresses of life." (Source: APA Dictionary of Psychology).

Roles must be assumed by all in fostering the positive mental health of residents.

The Role of Fellow Residents

Fellow residents play a key role in our day-to-day lives. Connecting with residents can take many forms: a friendly wave of "hello" across the room, gabbing together with twin wheelchairs, reaching for the hand of someone looking sad, cheering for another's evident progress, a sincere compliment, and a smile as big as the ocean! These can increase a fellow resident's confidence and energy level and reduce stress and anxiety.

Conversations with residents can be described as easy banter. We talk about our health and age to get to know one another. Like those who are not seniors, we discuss whatever we can remember that seems relevant to the conversation. No one seems to speak to impress, only to inform.

> *"There are no strangers here, only friends you haven't yet met." William Butler Yeats*

The Role of Roommates

Coexisting with a roommate is a key component of resident life. We must focus on the positives of such relationships: companionship, mutual support, and a greater chance to accept resident life.

During my months-long stay, I've had several roommates, each very different. First, there was Roommate 1, a very nice, quiet and unassuming person. Then came effervescent Roommate 2, a good conversationalist. When you called her name, she responded loudly, "WHAT??" seemingly indignant for having been disturbed. So full of vim and vigor!

Then I lived with Roommate 3, an intermittent resident who didn't waste time with niceties; she had strong opinions. Roommate 4 had worked for over 40 years at the same company, respected everyone, and tried not to make any waves. Roommate 5 spent her last weeks in pain and mostly alone.

My current roommate, Roommate 6, is an educated woman with unparalleled manners yet an unpredictable memory. "Since my stroke," she'll say. She is my sounding board and always has time to listen to another hot-off-the-press piece I've written. I am grateful to her. As a fellow resident, she can substantiate what I write about us residents and the workings of the facility.

I know this: I've learned from each of my roommates during their stay with me at this facility. One must be a good sport, accept the idiosyncrasies any roommate brings, and always try to be kind, understanding, and helpful. Just do it! Remember that you may not be the easiest person to live with!

The Role of Family and Friends

You are our penultimate champions and advocates, which means that the support and love you give us are secondary only to that offered by God!

"Walk a Mile in My Shoes" (Joe South), or with boots or braces—please try to! And not with pity but with understanding, patience, and encouragement.

Note to all: Friends and family, tending to an infirm loved one, even occasionally, is at some cost to their own, often hectic, lives. Their devotion only serves to remind us of their support and love.

I have always thought of love not as an amount but as a process of doing a series of good things. Our most cherished ones visit, arrange for snacks to be delivered, pick up a much-needed item (a new brush, notebook, or tee-shirt), send photos, bring flowers, phone us, text, or send emails, and pay our bills. They do all this, though it may disrupt their own non-stop responsibilities, obligations, and routines. It is not so easy to cater to the ongoing needs of an aging or disabled individual.

For those who may wonder at the frequency or infrequency of the support they provide, I say only the resident is to judge the contributions of the heart and the impact they make on our well-being. We appreciate the time spent with us and on our behalf; we do not expect a daily vigil from our friends and family! For the most part, simply knowing of their continuing thoughts and prayers for progress goes a long way. That support is immeasurable. We love them and appreciate their many gifts. I often turn to John Denver's "Perhaps Love" for an all-encompassing look at love.

Telephone Visits

Except for my teen years, I've disliked communicating by phone. This is similar to how my mom and dad felt about phone communication: I don't know why. It's good that no former job depended solely upon that to fulfill job responsibilities. Now, however hungry to hear your voice, I ask that you call, and we'll have a great chat!

The Nursing Staff, the Heart of Any Facility.

Nurses are the heart of any Skilled Nursing Facility. I wrote the following to honor the nursing staff here. Sadly, it has not been shared with them until now!

Note: Honoring the Nursing Staff on National Nurses' Day, May 6, 2024

> *Who cares about all that we have faced and probably still do? Who tries to help with all of that? Who is it that we can turn to - on almost an hourly basis for comfort? Who will hold our hand?*

The Residents: The Centerpiece of Any Facility

Today, May 6, 2024, is National Nurses' Day; we will celebrate National Nurses' Week all week.

After all of the aforementioned "Imaginings" I shared with you, what or who is it that rescues us? Who recognizes that although our bodies have deteriorated and are not in the best shape, our hearts still beat (with love, mostly), and our brains and minds still think? Our great spirit still sings! We are alive! Who cares that it is so? Who comes running when we call?

During the 18 months I have resided at this facility, I have come to know the nurses and the nursing/care staff at large, as well as the physical therapists, housekeepers, and even a social worker or two.

A Toast to You, Our TLC-Givers!

You have experienced the "Imaginings" mentioned at the beginning and have dealt with each of them admirably, in the most professional, caring, and supportive ways.

You have established a "medication routine," keeping the agonizing pain at bay! We respect your knowledge of medicine and caregiving.

You fulfill the slightest but most important requests: Please open and close my window, hand me my Kleenex, get another box of Kleenex, pull the shade up (or down), water the flowers, turn on my fan, pick out something from the closet to wear, find my phone, get the TV remote from the floor, etc., etc.!

You know how to work the machines and gadgets that make some mobility possible: the Hoyer, wheelchair, easy lift, and slide board. You do so without grumbling or complaining.

You, who provide the most care to the residents, are also our chief supporters, cheerleaders, and comforters. We honor you and your never-ending, forever assistance and love.

We thank you for dealing with indelicate matters concerning basic human needs.

We cherish each of you and your much-needed, cheery hellos and thoughtful comments: "How are you today? I thought of you last night after our conversation." "Would you like me to call your daughter for you?" "I don't have you on my list of residents to care for today, but I wanted to see how you're doing." "I like that color on you!" "When you first came here, you couldn't do anything." "You're doing great now." (making progress).

We delight in your stories about your families and life experiences. We love to laugh with you. We miss you when you are not here and when you go far away. We simply value you.

We effortlessly honor you today. Thank you for choosing the giving of "care" as your line of work and your calling. You are our fortress and light.

Sincerely,

Sonja Schmieder

Here is my list of the Top 30 nurses and aides on 2 West. It includes outstanding caregiving traits and habits to be emulated. I consider each of them a friend and part of my extended family.

"My friends are my estate." (Emily Dickinson)

The Residents: The Centerpiece of Any Facility

Rosaline: Rosie is my mainstay; she knows me as well as anyone. She is my caregiver and my confidant. We have traveled this long road together, with laughter and through tears. Steady as she goes! I want more for her and ask much of her: to assume a leadership role, one she can do well and naturally.

May and My T.: The nursing profession is lucky to have two outstanding representatives! They care first and foremost about the residents and the care each one is entitled to. On their respective shifts, we are confident that someone is in charge and making good decisions.

My T.: I simply cherish you.

May, my friend, has such a strong work ethic. Her oversight of the aides requires each one to do an all-encompassing job and to do it well! She is always "on," and her feet never stop moving. I appreciate her organization and wisdom, and I see the depth of her caring.

Twenty-two months ago, these three besties (Rosie, May, and My T.) welcomed a pathetic-looking and constantly-in-pain new resident into their care—me. I could never have made the evident strides without their professional know-how and skill. Their contributions to my health and well-being are immeasurable; their kindness and compassion are never-ending. Their stories and ideas always lift my spirits. I love them and thank them.

Fred is a hands-on nurse manager who spends much of his time with residents, tending to their large and small needs. Nothing is beneath him or his dignity. You can catch him delivering breakfast trays, accompanying doctors on their visits, and giving status reports at care conference meetings. He is the go-to guy on floor 2!

Mercy has left this facility, but I will always hold her close. She told it like it was, never letting anyone interfere with what was rightfully due to any resident.

Her good friend Cynthia is bright and competent and can also shake up the place if things are not done correctly.

Oretha is my overnight aide; she makes me feel safe. We talk and disturb the ominous quiet.

Two outstanding aides, Medina and Teagan, are up-and-coming nurses who are made for the job! At only 24 and 18 years old, respectively, they know instinctively what the job requires and are eager to learn more. They carry themselves well, with grace and humility.

The A-Team, Frances and Fredrick: Both are capable and experienced individuals who have worked as aides for many years. They are good-hearted and go out of their way to please all residents and fulfill their needs and requests. They also use humor to lighten things up!

Hamid and Vincent: Tracking everything related to dispensing the proper medications at the right time is a huge responsibility and should not be taken lightly. Plus, as with May and My T, there are regular interruptions. These interruptions include residents' questions that only "the nurse" can answer and procedures only the nurse can perform. This keeps everybody hopping and putting huge numbers of steps on their pedometers! Thanks to Hamid for helping me with tech questions and supporting my book.

Martha: Should operating a specific apparatus require two aides, or does carrying out a particular task require another assistant? Martha is the one to call! She can distribute meals, attend to her residents, and be quiet until she has questions!

Joseph: He is such a sweet and kind person. Happy to help!

Heather: Heather's laughter and morning greetings have us saying, "Hello again, World!" This strong-willed, Irish-looking lass is always ready to assist anyone. Just put your light on, and she's there, whether or not you are assigned to her.

Selena: Selena does her work effectively, efficiently, and expediently! We have great talks and are of the same political persuasion and beliefs.

Patti: She is the No-Nonsense Nurse! Behind that demeanor, she has a heart of gold. Great wit!

Stephan: He comes in to save any shift short of help!

Jackie: Jackie is fast on the draw, quick to assess and act to fix a situation. She is the first to answer anyone's call light. She goes out of her way to fulfill residents' requests.

Axel: Axel is the nicest and kindest of the lot! He makes each of us feel like we matter. He's also a member of the National Guard, serving his country but away from us for months at a time.

Eric: We sometimes have to borrow Eric from the third floor, which delights us. He is so good at his job and so lovely to be around.

Nemo: I can't remember Nemo ever questioning or hedging a request from a resident or staff member. She is always on it, determined to follow through to fulfillment.

Marpue: A careful start to our eventual and solid friendship! She is an exemplary caregiver and one who always encourages progress.

Travis: A veteran whose faith informs thoughtful decisions about resident care; he treats residents and coworkers respectfully and has a great sense of humor.

SamSam and Ann: Your quick visits to say hello and ensure all is well are welcomed and appreciated; you are good souls.

Maria: This Nurse Practitioner's pointed questions about residents' health are balanced by her deep gratitude for all things great and small and her ever-colorful wardrobe.

Favour: "Stay out of my way!" Favour is a gem in the making! She knows what to do and how to do it! Watching her soar!

Ingrid: This nurse sees it all! She is quick to move on to anything demanding attention.

To others who work on this floor: You, too, are essential in this critical undertaking. Residents only survive with the assistance and attention each of you provides.

And so, to each of you, and in the words of the insightful poet Maya Angelou,

The Residents: The Centerpiece of Any Facility

"I have learned that people will forget what you said, people will forget what you did, but people will never forget how you made them feel."

I will never forget.

Relationship-Building at the Facility

Building such relationships boosts our self-confidence and self-esteem and simply makes us happy.

The relationships we establish are essential to fostering our good mental health. Ongoing interactions with those closest to us and new friends or acquaintances can make for a good or bad day. Relationships are the glue that helps keep us together.

Isn't almost everything of importance about people and how they interact with each other? Here, we must emphasize the importance of an organization's ability to build and sustain close relationships. These are personal and professional relationships with and among residents, their family members and friends, co-workers, and the community.

The goal is to aid in the well-being of all within the facility. Relationship-building is fundamental to an SNF's success. Trusting relationships involve learning, listening, caring, and sharing interactions; they are built across the board, and everyone feels their positive effects. All who practice openness, honesty, and respectfulness allow such relationships to thrive, boosting a facility's likelihood of accomplishment.

In this intentionally built environment, everyone is a part of the group and belongs! Each person contributes something to the group, even if it is only their presence or the occasional moan or murmur, as with the frailest residents. Regardless of the contribution level, the group accepts each person and considers each a bona fide member.

Nurses and Short-Staffing Issues

How can a floor be continually short of staff? Are there no rules governing such practices? All too often, shifts are short-staffed, which puts an extra burden on caregivers to attend to the needs of more residents than the number usually on their daily list. This shortage can result in staff feeling overwhelmed and residents being shortchanged for attention.

The number of residents a nurse must care for may need to be lowered. When nurses are short-staffed, they have to cater to the needs of not only their regular number of residents but also the needs of others assigned from the lists of employees who have yet to show up for work. A resident may ask for something to be done and be refused. This situation may cause resentment toward the resident for making the request rather than toward a member of management for not anticipating the possible problem in the first place! This puts everyone in an untenable position.

Questions of Concern:
- Why must residents wait until we are four hours into a shift to find out who our on-duty aide is or to talk with them? A courtesy greeting to all on the list of individual

nurses at the beginning of each shift would be a nice, comforting gesture. One idea is for residents to use their call lights to greet the new shift, but call lights should only be used as a call for help.

- If we cannot tidy our rooms, could someone please help us? We live in a confined space that is best kept pleasing and presentable.
- We've had such beautiful weather! Why is there never time for residents to be outside for fresh air and sun? Patio, anyone?
- Can we please keep the water and the waste basket within reach?
- Could volunteers help with these things?

New Nurses/Aides

Many new young faces are on the floor; some are immediately impressive in their work, while others are not as interested or dedicated to the cause. What effect has their training had in causing such a distinction?

Note to Nurses' Aides: What traits will residents and their families value most in a nurse or an aide? What kind of nurse do you want to be?

Recruits are assumed to have received instruction (or experience) in caring for and working with the elderly and infirm.

Beyond that, keeping in mind their basic training about what to do and how to do it (that's a ton!), here's a quick checklist of questions, perhaps a few not yet considered. These items can be for new nurses' aides to ask themselves, as well:

- What do you know about the long-term resident on your care list this morning, this afternoon, or tonight?
- Briefly, what is their condition or disorder?
- How will your mood affect any interaction between you and those residents on your list?
- How well can the resident communicate with you?
- How mobile are they? Can they turn? Sit up? Walk?
- Are they tender in spots that require careful attention or avoidance? Given that information, what are your expectations of them while in your care?
- How might you help with their hair?
- Can you get them a washcloth to wash their face?
- Do they need you to get anything they cannot reach? TV remote, a blanket or sweater, a fan, toothbrush and paste, books, a can of pop from the cabinet, a new box of Kleenex, or hand wipes? Do they need lotion on their back or legs?
- Is their call light within reach? Is the phone charger plugged in?
- Will they be sitting in their wheelchair today?
- How do they get into the chair, by hoyer or slide board? For how long, approximately? Will you need to get them back into bed before your shift ends?
- Are condiments on the meal tray? A few extras?

- Do they have fresh water handy?
- Are all supplies you used put back into the resident's drawer and not left on the resident's meal tray?
- Were all items to be laundered labeled and bagged and taken out of the resident's room?
- Are residents going outside the facility today?
- Though they can call you, how often should you check on residents during your shift? They may need to ask a question of a nurse, a social worker, a PT, or the ride scheduler.
- At the end of your shift, ask yourself how the residents in your care benefited, what you can report about them that is significant, or what you will remember about them for the next time to help you establish your care routine for them. Thank you!

The Role of Management in Fostering Positive Mental Health

From my vantage point, I see many in management removed from residents' daily lives—other than greeting them "hello" or discussing financial matters. Greater involvement would foster goodwill and better mental health.

Here are some ideas on how Skilled Nursing Facilities can be crucial in promoting good mental health. These suggestions aim to bridge the gap between caregivers and management, fostering collaboration to support residents. Additionally, they explore opportunities to engage others in facility happenings to connect with residents.

Many suggestions emphasize using small group discussions facilitated by experts. Let's do it!

Engage and Empower

Involve residents in different ways in the daily life of the facility and the community. Find ways for residents to feel useful. Lying in bed all day and all night does little to stimulate the brain. Our brains are naturally quite active but might sometimes need an extra push. If not, we can become complacent and easily demoralized.

Many residents, through observations alone, can tell you a more effortless and better way to make facility operations run smoothly. For example, making mealtime run more effectively and dealing more tactfully with peer issues or conflicts.

Residents can tell you which people/nurses are most effective at their jobs, especially how they treat others, including their coworkers. They can tell you how that treatment reflects their feelings about their careers. Never interpret near silence as deadness.

The Value of Residents' Experience

Life is a series of experiences. As older adults, we've had many life experiences, some good, some not. We have learned from our experiences and have some knowledge to pass on to anyone who might benefit from it. What has each of us learned that we might share with others? Our experiences can foster awareness and understanding of similar situations or events in others' lives.

Think of the time you spent on the soccer field or the balance beam; the time you spent learning to play a musical instrument, driving a car, or studying to reach an understanding of biology or chemistry.

Think about the one who broke your heart and the perfect-for-you one who followed; about the job you loved where things went well, the one where not much went your way (but oh, did you learn what not to like!); think about the people you've met, and how "stand-out's" influenced your life.

We must not so easily dismiss a lifetime of learning. There are appropriate times when such learning begs to be shared so that others might have an easier, more knowledgeable path to follow. Might you have something to share about the knowledge you gained from your hard-fought experiences? Think you know yourself, your subject? Might you want to share what you've learned with those who might be receptive to the information?

It's our time to share!

Many residents in any facility like this could recall some of the experiences, expertise, and wisdom gained from their work or home lives. This knowledge could and should be utilized and shared with others. How can we tap into that treasure trove? How can we make that happen?

Residents need to be included in the decision-making process; being of sound mind, I, for one, resent not being asked what I think about anything related to my life!

Getting Residents to Open Up

Improve the facility by incorporating residents' know-how and past experiences. Beyond voicing complaints, a skilled facilitator can conduct small group discussions about how to do so, e.g., "What are your ideas to make things here run more smoothly?" Give an example: "We need to…"

Putting residents' minds to "work" on some concern or problem would do wonders for their mood, which can have positive physical effects. More than a handful of residents might find this both refreshing and invigorating.

Let's Talk About Our Feelings

Small group interactions can help uncover, express, or even vent the feelings of many residents. Use a prepared list of questions to begin such discussions slowly and carefully, e.g., "Today I feel like…" Set a time limit on responses to each question. Ask what the facility can do to alleviate feelings of anxiety or stress.

Some residents love to read. How about discussions centered around a particular book, passages from a book, or discussions about a poem? Or having a real author make a presentation of their book?

Resident Council Meetings

Many SNFs have residents gather monthly at a Resident Council Meeting or assembly to provide input on pertinent matters or simply to voice complaints about something unacceptable to them. However, attendance at opportunities to voice concerns may be sparse, as some residents may be too sick to attend, making their participation impossible. Others may not feel comfortable speaking out in front of any size group—and, in their past lives, have seldom done so—while some may be too shy to ask a question.

By the way, many of these same people will approach those brave enough to speak up or those with effective speaking and presentation skills to say they were glad the speakers asked those questions or made that statement because they feel the same way about the topic. No matter how practiced and courageous the speakers are, support is always most appreciated when comments are made!

I attended my first meeting in the Chapel, where about 15 people sat in a circle, each looking over the planned agenda.

The items for discussion, led by the Council's President, addressed new and old business concerns including food services, activities, administrative updates, comments about the nursing staff, laundry/housekeeping issues, and a review of "the confidentiality of residents' records."

The minutes from Council Meetings should be shared with all residents so that all residents know what has transpired.

The Use of Volunteers

I suggest drafting a new plan to recruit volunteers - neighbors and church members - who would bring new life into the facility. This decision would tap into the kindness of those of all ages in the neighborhood, and those church-affiliated organizations would bring life to the facility. They could be facilitators of the exercises suggested above. Or, they might enhance the facility's offerings. Volunteers could serve coffee, tea, and snacks around 3:30-ish, welcome faces in playing board games with residents, add their voices to sing-alongs, and be partners in residents' hobbies, including all things sewing and craft-related.

Community Involvement

Furthermore, there are community events and happenings (besides Twins games) that residents could participate in and contribute to. For those able to do so, being part of the wider community would help residents feel somewhat normal. Shopping for flowers, anyone? Helping to staff a community booth?

Beyond Viewing Our Favorite TV Shows

Could we use the channel hookup, which broadcasts weekly Bible study lessons for presentations made to residents when part of the facility is shut down due to an outbreak of one or two cases of COVID-19? This could foster community when all group activities have been temporarily canceled.

Could we add more activities that involve exercise and fresh air? These two things are essential for the health of the elderly. Ah, to breathe again (or learn to breathe again)! To work out (even a bit)!

> **Teachers Facilitate Learning:**
> **The Involvement of Educators**
>
> How about this? A secret solution to eliciting what residents know and—when feeling better—can contribute. This suggestion involves the possible participation of our teaching and retired teaching forces to cooperate, coordinate, and work side-by-side with healthcare professionals. This kind of partnership could result in unearthing residents' knowledge (stories), fears, backgrounds, life lessons, values, and the like.
>
> Teachers are experts at teaching and conveying information. They know how to motivate people; they are good at staging non-threatening learning environments. Teachers are experts at asking the right questions and getting desired feedback, and they are well-versed in challenging people to do something, do more, and never give up! They are ideal attitude changers; in this case, they would be excellent at fostering positive attitudes to deal with change, illness, and expectations. They are ready to help, and are sensitive and empathetic, making them ideal candidates to work with the sick and elderly. Perfect facilitators!
>
> Teachers will find ways to engage those seated in the dining room who are quietly waiting for their meal. For example, devise a "Today's Big Question," a mini-puzzle, for each grouping to discuss; select a moderator and note-taker at each table to report answers. This is for thoughts that come to mind

> quickly and from anyone—it's not complicated. Do you have other ideas?
>
> They could develop an information-gathering process for feedback by eliciting feedback from residents through survey questions, focus group discussions, one-on-one interactions, questionnaires, mini-interviews, and observations.
>
> These kinds of strategies could indicate what works best with residents from their point of view. They would help strengthen any decisions made, as the pool of expertise would be significantly widened. There would be less grousing behind closed doors.

Mental Health: A Couple of Personal Issues

As a resident of this facility, I am learning more about myself as others learn more about themselves.

1. I've learned that I am a sprinter. Ask me to run a marathon or do almost anything over too long a distance, and I become impatient to move on. Do you see the problem in being confined to long-term care? It requires a strong, steady, and hopeful frame of mind. "Mind over matter," they say. "Just wait it out!"

   At the outset, my family figured my stay at this facility might be weeks. At this point, I was not fixated on the time I'd have to spend here. Was I just too sick to be preoccupied with thoughts of moving on, or had I finally developed some patience? Now that I've made so much progress in my physical health and shown a vast improvement in mobility, I'm again feeling discontent. "I'm out of here!" screams and streams out of me.

2. Where am I at this stage of my life? I know that I am loved. But, looming large is the not-so-wonderful and stark realization that I need, yet I am not needed. How on earth is it possible for others to do well without me, without my help? *"They might not need me, but they might." (Emily Dickinson).*

This is mind-blowing! It has caused me to rethink the reason for my existence. I must accept this truth/challenge/change. I try to!

It makes me wonder what it will be like when no one wants me in their homes, at their gatherings, or their tables.

"For who can bear to feel himself forgotten?"
W.H. Auden

Strength to Stand

4

Management: Orchestrating Care

The residents are the centerpiece of any facility. The nurses and nursing staff are at the heart of any Skilled Nursing Facility, and management makes the decisions.

Background

During my "salad days" (which, amazingly, lasted for years), I worked at various times for seven nonprofit 501(c)(3) education associations at their headquarters in Washington, DC, and Minnesota. This followed nine years of teaching the best-ever third graders! I was once asked in a job interview, "What's the longest you've held a job?" because the duration of most nonprofit programs and projects was only three or four years each.

My work at these associations centered on planning and managing educational and staff development programs and projects for teachers, school principals, and educators in higher education across the country. The goal was to inform them about innovative educational improvement initiatives and encourage participation. All were funded by dues from members of the organizations, grants from federal and/or state governments, or private-sourced monies.

These programs and projects offered participants various training and retraining opportunities. They brought the latest in educational research to educators at all levels. They sparked new thinking in teaching and learning strategies and highlighted the best, most successful teaching and education practices. It caused those involved to form strong and long-lasting networks and to share classroom successes, all before social media.

Students are at the core of any educational endeavor. The goal was to ensure that opportunities like these afforded to participating educators would give students a greater chance to acquire the knowledge, skills, and attitudes necessary to become fully functioning members of a global society.

Here's the point: I am now a resident of a 501(c)(3). Life is strange that way! My observations here help me recall my time working in a nonprofit world. I can readily spot areas of weakness and causes for concern and, therefore, respectfully point out possible refinements for improvement.

This facility has been my home for 22+ months. I know most of the nursing staff on this floor quite well. I know a few on the management side, but very little about them. I am removed from these individuals by space, as management resides on a different floor. I have also been removed from them over time, as almost none of them spend quality time with residents daily.

I am detached, for the most part, from the work that they do. I suppose this makes it easier to blame or complain when things do not run smoothly. Management runs the place, and if things are not working well or as well as they should, the fault can naturally reside there.

I am not an employee of the facility; therefore, I am free to speak up or sound off about matters relating to the facility's operation, especially when those issues affect the lives, health, or general well-being of the residents and staff.

This Skilled Nursing Facility is good— it has the potential to be great!

When input is requested about hot topics at this nonprofit, I might have some information to add that will improve the situation, even if it is only a respectful suggestion on how to do something better.

My experience in education and nonprofit organizations and working in program implementation provide a unique, perhaps even valuable, perspective regarding the programs, leadership, management, staff, and residents here.

Key Management Roles

It would be helpful for every family to know key management officials as well as options offered to residents by the Physical and Occupational therapy department, food services and social workers. All are integral to the overall care and support residents receive, and are subject to service assessments and satisfaction reports.

Outstanding management practices apply to parent company executives, as well.

Sample questions for parent company executives:

> How does information flow to you from your facilities?
>
> How many members of staff do you work directly and frequently with—and know well—at each of your facilities?
>
> Do you know about and care what services residents living at your facilities are missing out on?
>
> How well do you know the needs of your facilities—needs that, when satisfactorily fulfilled, could positively alter the very lives of residents?
>
> What new ideas have you recently implemented to make life easier for residents and staff—ideas that are innovative, fun, and could be widely shared among your facilities?
>
> Who are your go-to leaders whose leadership might be emulated?
>
> How do the state's star ratings align with your interpretation of the work done by your facilities?

Board of Directors

The Board of Directors is the governing body of the 501(c)(3) nonprofit organization. Know who the members of the Board of Directors are of the nonprofit facility you are looking at, and get a snapshot of their backgrounds. Understand how Board members are selected, as well as their roles and responsibilities, such as helping to fulfill the organization's mission, conducting community outreach, fundraising, providing financial oversight, and having knowledge of nonprofit laws and regulations. The Board is in the organization's prime leadership position and is responsible for making decisions that affect the organization's accountability and degree of success.

Managers

So many people in management and staff positions care so much about doing their jobs well. These individuals possess a strong and impressive work ethic, often honed over many dedicated years. They know they bring value to their organizations, schools, companies, corporations, or entrepreneurial endeavors. For their efforts, they may be lauded in different ways, i.e., a raise in salary, special work perks, award plaques, notes of appreciation, good press, and social celebrations. They revel in their accomplishments and the sure knowledge that by doing their "piece of the puzzle" and doing it well, they add value to their respective institutions.

Management

A core responsibility of top management is to support the facility's people, including the residents, staff, and fellow managers. Despite good intentions, this priority may slide when top managers become overwhelmed by weighty matters and paperwork demands.

Management deals with conflict within the organization, between and among residents, between residents and staff, and within management itself. Conflict is natural; a strong, careful, tactful, and diplomatic manager can resolve disputes in any stressful environment, but dealing with older, sick, and sometimes discouraged residents—and those who work with them—can be challenging, to say the least!

Where do increases in wages and bonuses fit into the picture of growing a more effective organization and building morale? What about promotions and other advancements? Why is no one allowed to talk about that?

Other Nonprofits

As a new employee, I remember being immediately introduced to management's key individuals and encouraged to call upon them whenever the situation warranted. Why this "open-door" policy? It creates an atmosphere that indicates we are all working together to make the organization as strong and effective as possible. There always seemed to be "top brass" members stopping by to ask questions or visit. They made the time for that! In doing so, they sent a message that our opinions were valued and that we were contributing to the wealth and health of the organization. Because we were informed about how and what individuals in departments were doing, there were fewer surprises or causes for panic.

Communication: An Essential Skill of Management

Today, we met the facility's new Administrator. This happened by chance because he was making a few rounds and stopped in to attend my care conference. I was happy to have him participate in the discussion. I hope there are more formal plans

Management: Orchestrating Care

to welcome him and some "press" about his background and credentials, as he is now in a key leadership position here.

We want to know who this person is at the helm and what his plan is for implementing the organization's mission. A special flier, social gathering, perhaps?

It is good for residents and their families to know who comes and goes at this facility. We need to understand how best to contact those now in authority (email, phone, floor nurse, etc.). For those who are no longer with the facility, we are still interested in their whereabouts and doings.

The Website

In today's world, where so much of our lives revolve around using the Internet, I recommend that this facility consider updating and sprucing up its website. It likely gives prospective residents, their families, and friends a first impression. The website should provide information and photos about the site's mission, offerings, unique features, ratings, and reviews. It should also contain pictures of board members, key management and staff members, and residents, showing their engagement in fun activities.

The website should reflect the ambiance of the facility and highlight why selecting this facility over another might be a good choice. It should also include a comments section featuring critiques from those who have experienced life at the facility—as residents, family members, management, or staff—as each might see things differently.

Communicating With Residents

Communication with residents has improved. Notices of upcoming meetings and activities are posted in the elevators, and fliers are handed out to residents in their rooms. Announcements continue throughout the PA system, although most cannot be heard well in residents' rooms.

In case of when the first alarm goes off as a drill or in an emergency, we need someone to immediately inform residents of the seriousness of the situation instead of closing each resident's room door without explanation. We must also know the protocol for correct conduct and procedures during a fire or severe weather.

I prefer Mary Ann's best communication method, a brief visit to remind residents in each room of an event or Bible study group session that will be happening within the hour. This reminder's timing is easy for residents to remember and provides a chance to exchange a few words with her.

Newsletter

I would like to see a short newsletter distributed occasionally quoting residents' answers to questions such as: What do you like most about this facility? Who are your closest friends here? What are you watching on TV? Any news you'd like to share about your grandchildren? What do you remember about raising your children, i.e., what worked well? Where have you traveled? Most tremendous honor or pleasure you've received? What is your favorite book or movie? Favorite song, singer? Etc. Quotes could be posted on the website.

Management: Orchestrating Care

We residents draw comfort from seeing the same friendly faces who come to care for us on a regular basis. We grow attached to them, as they develop their own style of care suitable for each resident assigned to them.

To augment bits of news found in The Perk or the Daily Brief, I would like to see a "For Your Information" (FYI) section in the newsletter that would inform residents why certain individuals from the nursing staff we are used to seeing on their regular shifts are missing:

1. We will miss —and —, who have gone "back home" for a few months' visit; have fun!
2. —and —are no longer on 2West; they have chosen instead to care for family members in their respective homes.
3. —has moved on to another SNF. Who will greet us each morning with a cheery "hello?"
4. The resident doctor, Dr. —, has been replaced by Dr. —.

A Note to Residents: Oftentimes, nurses or aides choose not to share their plans with residents, fearing it might cause distress. However, without this information, we are left to wonder, feel uncertain about our care, and even worry that something has gone wrong. That uncertainty is the worse choice.

In the end, not to worry, as others on staff have stepped in to try to fill the void, and new people continue to come on board.

Feedback

Sometimes, we know too little about the people we interact with so closely every day. And we know even less about those who work on different floors. Is it too "old school" to encourage using a Suggestion Box for residents to anonymously drop in suggestions for specific changes that would upgrade the facility and its workings? A place to offer a vote for a resident of the month or a staff member of the month? A place where residents could read write-ups about fellow residents and staff to learn more about their work and families? Maybe even see photos of those being honored?

Nurses: On the Frontline

As one nurse told me, "I walk the floors." Walk with me and see what needs to be done. Only when you are in the throes of resident life can you make the most prudent and accurate decisions that, at the most basic level, affect the very lives of older people!

Walking these floors would reveal less than prudent decision-making: staff (many of them are recruits) call to say they will not be coming in repeatedly or that they have quit, leaving gaping holes in the effectiveness of an organization that is a competent one. Other staff members on shift are told to make do and to add "extra" residents to their already overwhelming workload. Nurses can be asked to oversee 25-50 patients per shift. Do you see a danger in that?

This facility needs to examine all these issues carefully and thoroughly. A good facility like this one is at an inflection point, and some critical issues must be addressed sufficiently and immediately. One of the main issues is the mind-blowing expectations for staff, specifically the day-shift staff. There are also issues of staff and management turnover, a shortage in food services, morale concerns, gaps in training, and scarcity of significant supplies.

Morale

What about the morale of those in management? There are individuals in management whose primary job is to (try to) manage one area of importance by themselves; they may feel overwhelmed at the responsibility thrust upon them!

Training

There are spaces to fill in staff training, such as using a slide board, explaining how to help residents learn to walk again, providing tips for changing diapers and using equipment, and providing overviews of residents' conditions that contribute to an understanding of the kind of care required, and more.

Is there a system that concentrates on the needs of the facility's residents and the nursing staff who care for them?

Management, take the walk! Do more than greet residents; sit with the nurses attending them for a while. Be prepared to learn!

See your expectations for staff and whether the expectations and demands are feasible! Know the degree of care required by each resident, and know how best to understand the staff workload and how to divide it. Take the time to develop a plan to fill in any observable gaps in the care and support system. Consider how the information gleaned might aid in recruiting and retaining nurses and the nursing staff.

Management: Financial Matters

The Healthcare System

Upon entering any healthcare facility, following an obligatory "Hello, how are you today?" greeting, you will be asked, "Do you have your insurance card(s) with you?"

Translated, this means: If you wish to see this particular person or if we do this procedure, who will pay for it?

Finances

Paying Skilled Nursing Facilities: "We don't provide free care and support services to long-term residents." Why not? Eventually, if we live long enough, we all need long-term care. If one has to be in such a facility, why must we spend every cent of what we have saved or receive in monthly pay (Social Security and other benefits) to be "housed" in an SNF? Why must we be left with little to spend or to help out our families? Why must we let the people who never went after the big money and only "served" others lose everything as they deal with sickness, disease, or a rare condition?

Management: Orchestrating Care

First and foremost, please know that the level or quality of care does not define a facility and its many necessary parts. However, care is a critical component of the operation in general. What matters most is profitability—even for a nonprofit—so that the organization can continue to exist and that any "extra" funds can be used to broaden the services offered by the facility.

I am, most fervently, taking on the fight for a healthcare system that begs to be more user-friendly, effective, and efficient. One where care is on a par with profits. A system that supports care facilities and their people. A system and a country that provides for its elderly, their families, and those who care for them.

We cannot just advocate for good and affordable healthcare for all. We must develop and adopt principles, rules, and regulations that are understandable, fair, and workable for clients/customers/residents thrust into a system they know little or nothing about. The present system is almost unnavigable, especially for those who have yet to experience the insanity of a redundant system that is neither transparent nor acceptable.

The care of and for residents cannot be a secondary factor in the overall system. It must be put first, and the hunger for profits must follow.

Working with the State & County on Medical Assistance

As you try to navigate the system, particularly in seeking medical assistance for long-term care and helping to cover expenses incurred at your selected facility, please consider the following:

The Application

In addition to the requisite information about you, such as your name, gender, race, and U.S. citizenship, you will be asked questions about your living situation, financials/assets, insurance, employment, and medical expenses.

You will be asked for supporting documents with the option to upload directly to the County regarding such things as:

- Your checking account(s) balance(s) going back three or more months, including monies coming in (the amounts of any income such as Social Security and retirement benefits or pensions) and monies spent, including cash withdrawals or automated bill pay, as indicated by your monthly bank statements;
- Savings account (s) balance(s);
- Copies of Medicare and other insurance cards;
- Your life insurance information, precisely the cash value of your policy;
- Loans and transfers.

At this point, it's like standing naked, asking for financial help that might cover some of your expenses and being in a situation you'd rather not be in.

Once the application is received, there will be a waiting period—usually over a month—for the County to review it. As they conduct their review, they will ask for specific documents that inform the application review panel where your money has gone over the years. This ensures that you did not try to pull a fast

Management: Orchestrating Care

one, such as giving away monies, that might better be spent in payments to a Skilled Nursing Facility.

It is a challenging, complex world that expects you to work most of your life to build up your assets, only to declare them and watch them disappear to pay for "rent" at a "home" you did not build or choose. Ultimately, all this is so you can be as poor as a church mouse!

"*Gone Fishing*," sung by Chris Rae, says it all.

Working With the County

The County deals in facts and figures. There is little if any, human interaction involved in the process. This includes face-to-face meetings. You might be fortunate enough to reach someone in the County by phone for answers to questions. If you do, they may have questions for you as well. These questions are asked in a firm, no-nonsense manner by those holding your fate in their hands.

Be sure to request help navigating the system from the facility's social worker's office at the outset. Social workers are hired to help residents with their needs; they know the necessary resources and services available. Their work is confidential and guided by a Code of Ethics. Note: The social work department no longer assists with medical assistance applications at this facility.

You can also contact the County's Ombudsman Office for help. Their job is to protect residents' rights in long-term care and handle their complaints, grievances, and appeals. In general, they are a wealth of information about the healthcare system. At our facility, we have access to a traveling Ombudsman who covers several miles and several skilled nursing facilities. The Ombudsman becomes especially important to residents when the social workers do not provide assistance.

Note: When the Ombudsman stops by, you must be ready with your questions and have any necessary paperwork on hand. Advance notice would be nice that indicates his arrival and an estimated time for the length of the meeting. This short notice makes it almost impossible for a family member or lawyer to attend.

Should the review panel rule in your favor, you will receive medical assistance and the amount and specifics the County decides. Once a "pay schedule" is arranged, your allowance (to spend any way you wish) will be around $115 per month. Let's see, my cellphone—a real necessity, isn't it?—costs me $73 per month. $115 - $73 = not much left!

If your application is denied, you can submit another application. This whole process can be quite short or long and drawn out.

Update: My latest application for MA has been pending for over five months.

Medical Assistance: Some Specificity

In applying with the County for Medical Assistance, there may be no one to prepare you for what lies ahead or hold your hand while you try to understand how to work the system and what is being asked of you as you proceed. Only by denying your application will you finally learn the rules and jargon of how to do things correctly.

> In applying to the County, here are some things my family and I have learned about the Medical Assistance application:
> - The process begins with filling out a ten-page application. Simple enough, you think.
> - You wait for a reply from the County, which can be up to 45 days from applying.
> - You will receive a letter stating whether your application was accepted, denied, or pending until the requested documents are fully received.
> - You may be asked for even more detailed information about account expenditures for several years. Hopefully, you have kept your receipts! Any communication feels like it is done with a non-living entity like a building rather than a living, breathing County representative. It is done online; you upload the requested documents to InfoKeep.
> - Your case number must appear on all documents' front and back. Otherwise, documents or pages may be misplaced.
> - You are informed of any action taken regarding your case through US mail, which is a long haul.
> - If your application is denied (even several times) and you complain about the system and how it needs to be made more user-friendly, that's too bad. Social workers and the Ombudsmen will tell you, "It is the law," and "you must comply with it." They'll say the system is the same for everyone.

> - You will tear your hair out!

This all occurs over several months.

> *"If you don't like something, change it.*
> *If you can't change it, change your attitude."*
> *Maya Angelou*

Lessons Learned: Avoiding Potential Pitfalls

The following are some recommendations I have made to management, both in person and in writing. I am sharing them with you so that you will be ready to ask questions about essential pieces that can significantly enhance the nurturing of your loved ones at any SNF.

Raising Concerns

This special section aligns with the book's subtitle, *"Pulling Back the Curtain on Long-Term Care."* It highlights a long list of concerns compiled over many months and calls for management's attention. This section includes both letters and short shots.

Of course, everyone finds something troubling about any place where they spend significant time, whether it's a workplace, group setting, or residence.

The concerns expressed herein, including suggestions for adjustments or improvements, are meant to achieve excellence. They are not to be interpreted as an attempt to demean this establishment or to try to criticize specific members of management. Instead, it is an effort to name some of the operation's weaknesses or deficits and assist in finding ways to fix them.

Management: Orchestrating Care

In compiling such a list of separate concerns, I know that I was moving beyond mere dissatisfaction or annoyance about an issue or problem, having passed the stage of whining, griping, or grumbling. This is now the peaceful protest phase, and with no intention of filing a formal grievance.

Here, dear reader, are the stories behind the problems that I have personally experienced. Your mission is to take action on behalf of your loved one—or yourself—regarding any sudden troubles that may arise, impacting not only their physical well-being but also their emotional and mental health. We must speak up for residents who may face similar issues that require attention.

When management does not address, acknowledge, or outright ignores concerns, the message to residents is a loud, "You don't matter," or "I'm too busy to deal with that now." A better response would be, "Thank you! I received your message and will get back to you as soon as I can." This approach reassures the resident and prevents unnecessary fretting over the issue while giving the manager time to address and rectify the situation.

"What does the owl see tha the rest of the world is missing?" MJ Rose

Concern: Meals

For one's information: Three meals are served at this facility each day, at around 8:15 AM, 12:15 PM, and 5:15 PM. The lag between the last meal served at 5:15 PM and breakfast means residents can go without eating for 15 hours. There is no designated evening snack time or coffee served before breakfast. Would you be okay with such a routine?

Concern: Social Workers

The following stories recount my struggles to voice a concern and the steps involved in finding a solution to the problem.

The following excerpt is an addendum dated April 14, 2024, about the hit-and-miss involvement of social workers in my life/case at this SNF. New residents are, as a rule, assigned a social worker; however, the assignment of one does not ensure real back-and-forth interaction. And so, I wrote this to the administrator:

> *Dear —-,*
>
> *This provides additional testimony to reinforce that (during my tenure here), I have had very little interaction with any social worker. These individuals serve as liaisons between management, residents, and their families. They serve a critical role in the effectiveness and success of an SNF. They provide support and resources to residents beyond helping families understand and fill out required applications for financial assistance and transportation modes. They are professionals who abide by a strict code of ethics, value and practice resident confidentiality, and generally serve as a sounding board for residents; they can be a source of great comfort as residents and their families navigate the daunting health community system. They can, along with an assigned County Ombudsman, ensure that resident rights, e.g., "being free from verbal, sexual, physical, and mental abuse," are respected (State of Minnesota). Build an ongoing,*

working relationship with your social worker, as their involvement is invaluable and critical to an "easier" time spent at the facility.

February 8, 2024

Email to Facility Rep,

After our discussion yesterday about documents still outstanding in my application for Medicaid, as well as your comment about the length of time spent on my case, I've come to realize that (all along) in this process during my over a year's stay at this facility, how important it would have been to be working directly, over time, with a social worker, and preferably, the same one. This to help me deal with this undertaking and to be a bridge/advocate for my family.

There can't be many notes on file about my interactions/meetings with social workers here. I've reflected on any brief interactions with such persons, and this is what I recall:

1). Social Worker #1: She brought in a few breakfast trays, once came into my room with the head of the business office to request payment of my bill, and once came to my room to say I would have a care conference (now) in my room. She had a conversation several weeks ago that the Administrator knew about and apologized for, and one that ended with her walking out of my room in exasperation.

2). Social Worker #2: We had only one discussion. She said she would help me with the Medical Assistance paperwork but did not get back to me and then left the facility.

3). Social Worker #3: We had one conversation, followed by a productive meeting with my children, during which we were all hopeful of making progress regarding Medicaid. Then, she got sick for a few weeks, after which she called to ask why documents had not been sent to the County. I have not spoken to or seen her in the weeks since then.

4). Social Worker #4: He led my last care conference and submitted requested reports to include in my pending application to Courage Kenny for intensive therapy and rehabilitation.

A County Ombudsman assigned here gave me a list of people in the Minneapolis area who could help from the outside with paperwork and then declared he'd done everything he could for me and that, as far as he is concerned, my case is closed.

All to say, interactions with me by the individuals named above have not provided the time or emotional support I've needed to slog through this seemingly unending process.

Discussions with you recently have been productive; you've tried so hard to get things processed and in a timely manner, but I still have questions and concerns that a social worker should address.

This whole process has been a nightmare for my family. There is pressure to move things along as soon as possible, and some comments could have been more helpful instead of contributing to worry and angst.

Sonja

Update: The social work department has formed a new team! Things may be changing for the better!

Update 2: The department has lost two of their three new additions. It's time to reassess goals, duties, and incentives.

Concern: Transparency and Communication

We are forced to think and wonder about stuff. Most everything seems to be a big secret here, and no one is telling any secrets that could/should inform residents about what affects them or about something they've raised a concern about. Management should address this.

We residents sometimes need to know that management is aware of a problem and working on a solution. We need to know that management has taken the action we require, such as the possibility of assisted living or the availability of physical therapy, as promised. A quick PA announcement to allay concerns or fears would be welcomed.

Concern: Death & Dying

Dear Management,

I learned at 8:00 pm this evening that a fellow resident, one who resided across the hall, passed away last night. Had I not asked my aide how Gene is doing - as I have repeatedly done so during the past month - I would not have been told of his passing.

Gene and I had many discussions in the hall and by the window about almost any subject, particularly GM and Ohio, where he lived and worked - before he chose to confine himself to his room. He was well-spoken and knew a lot about a lot of things. He was an interesting conversationalist; when you reach ninety, there is plenty to talk about and many stories to share. He liked to look good and wear nice clothes. He was a determined walker with a small stash of treasures in his bin.

I feel sad and can't believe there is no means for fellow residents to learn about the fate of people they converse with regularly and that they get to know and care for.

Perhaps the new Pastor might make an announcement when this happens so that we residents can join him in saying a collective prayer to send the resident on his way with love.

There is nothing that needs to be kept confidential about someone dying. We need to show some respect and honor because that matters.

The same thing happened when Rosemary died. It was days later that someone spoke about it. Why would honoring people we have lived with be so difficult? Keeping that kind of information from fellow residents is cruel.

I, for one, will miss them both. They simply made life here more cheerful. Shooting the breeze with Gene was simply fun!

RIP, Friend.

Sonja Schmieder

Update: A resident passed away yesterday. Management arranged a "Walk of Honor," hosted by the new chaplain with prayers and songs. Another had his picture posted on the bulletin board announcing his passing. Appreciated.

Concern: The Use of MetroMobility

The State of Minnesota provides rapid, public transportation ("mini-buses") for riders of all ages with disabilities and other health concerns through its Metropolitan Council MetroMobility (MM). Fares for MetroMobility riders are much lower than those

Management: Orchestrating Care

charged by private companies. Its drivers are well-trained to assist riders when getting on and off the vehicles, and they know techniques for securing wheelchairs for those who need them, guaranteeing their safety.

Once I was approved to attend Courage Kenny as an outpatient, I sought information about using MetroMobility to travel to and from the Center. I had no idea that so much information, including some health history and proof of the prospective rider's disability, would be required to process the application. It makes sense!

I asked my facility for help getting the ball rolling. A social worker filled out the application form. A couple of weeks passed, and when I asked if he had heard anything regarding my application, he said, "Not yet." This implied that it was the MM office's next move.

I waited a week longer and then began calling the office myself to see whether my application had been received; it had not. I sought out the social worker who supposedly had submitted it and was told he would be away from the facility for a few weeks. A different social worker then checked for the application in the former's office, found it half-finished, and, with my help, completed it and faxed it to the state.

Another week went by. I checked a few times for receipt of the application, and still nothing was received. The second social worker called to see whether they had received the fax she sent, and as she was told they had not, she faxed the application. Another week went by.

As the weeks pass, I go to Courage Kenny for physical and occupational therapy appointments twice a week by private transport at $100 per ride.

Finally, I heard good news from the State Office: I have been approved to ride with MM, and they only need a photo ID. Because my driver's license expired during these past months, I had no existing photo ID. Once they received a new photo, they made an ID card for me and sent it along with a Go-To card to store my fare money.

I've been riding with MM for over a month. It is one of this state's grand achievements (among many!), as far as I can determine! Disabled persons pay a one-way fee of $3.50 ($7.00 per round trip) to attend Courage Kenny, doctor's appointments, or even a few social engagements.

I have seen parts of this glorious city I've never seen before, and I can visit with my kids and grandkids! Think of it! I can just sit back and relax, knowing that any of the many competent MM drivers has had extensive training in assisting disabled riders and in overall safety procedures. How incredible!

The above demonstrates that nothing can be taken for granted. Things must be checked and sometimes doggedly rechecked to ensure a good result. Be your own advocate or designate someone to follow through on such matters. I can fight for these things myself now, but there was a time when that was impossible. Think of the many elderly residents without anyone to untangle a mess or fight for them. Be one who does!

Concern: Seeing the Podiatrist

Yesterday, the messenger came to the room to announce that the podiatrist was here! Was I ready to go down? I was just about to leave the room to catch MetroMobility for another physical therapy appointment. I got a bit tetchy! (Not the messenger's fault!) I asked that this facility pay us the courtesy of letting us know the dates of the doctor's visits in advance so that we do not schedule another outside appointment at the same time. I needed to see the podiatrist because I had an infected nail that needed attention. Because I missed seeing him, I will have to wait another few months to be on the list again.

Today, I was told that the podiatrist and staff saw residents for only a few hours, then left the site, leaving many patients yet to be seen. Come on!

Update: The podiatrist did return for another visit; all was taken care of!

Concern: Laundry

Days ago, I sent down a new turquoise long-sleeved turtleneck to be labeled and washed. I have been asking for it for the past few days. The head of laundry and another worker could not find it. I was told to ask the aide who sent it down to be laundered where it might be (I don't know which aide did so.). It makes me a little wary, as months ago, I had to fill out a form for the loss of six pairs of workout pants, one pair of casual pants, and a t-shirt. It's maddening and seemingly neverending. Who in the world is keeping track of such goings-on for the residents?

Concern: Care Conferences

Tuesday, March 12, 2024

Dear Management,

This is to respectfully question the reasons for resident Care Conferences, any requirements for advance notice of conferences and agendas for same, invitees to conferences, and the sharing of outcomes of such conferences.

I was informed that my latest Care Conference was held today and was asked, "Didn't you want to attend?" I replied that I hadn't been notified it was scheduled and that, yes, I would have attended. Why? Because I am well enough to participate and eager to hear what people—and reports—say about my progress and any possible next steps toward my recovery.

Feedback to residents is critical. Care Conferences, which summarize months of health information, provide a serious and fair assessment, especially since visits from the attending physician and nurse practitioner are infrequent. Their visits often focus on questioning residents rather than incorporating insights from those directly involved in their care.

Today's failure to inform this resident is a big deal! Why? At my last Care Conference on December 21, 2023 (with the social worker as lead, and including Colin (PT), Sarah (Activities), and the nutritionist, I questioned why my family was not invited to attend (if only by phone or Zoom) so that they could hear of my status, first-hand. I asked further why my primary aide, Rosie, was omitted, as she works most closely and continuously with me. Conrad, who runs The Restorative Program, was also at the top of my list of suggested

Management: Orchestrating Care

attendees. Also, I asked that notes from the conference be shared with my family as they were not included in the conference; they were not sent to them.

In getting a fair assessment of a resident's health and progress, pulling information from all available (re)sources and sharing that information openly with all involved would provide a most accurate picture of each resident. Going the extra mile here can also help dispel any notion of conducting a quick Care Conference to check "done" on the State's requirements list. It would further paint a picture of what needs to be accomplished for the resident – goals to meet – by the next scheduled Care Conference.

In the future, what might be a plan for residents to know the dates of their conferences ahead of time (!) and the names of those who might best contribute to the overall picture of each resident? The conferences are vital to any Skilled Nursing Facility; they should not be taken lightly.

Sincerely,

Sonja Schmieder

Update: Yesterday, I received a note indicating that my next Care Conference will be in two weeks and that two family members are invited to attend in person and two others by phone! Speak up! People do listen!

Care Conferences should be held more often than every three or four months. Information about residents' health and progress should be shared as it is now. Still, it should also result in developing a plan for the future that defines expectations for the next few months leading up to the next Care Conference.

Note: Notes from Care Conferences are not currently shared with residents but are only on file with the nursing staff and social workers. How can residents and family members know the accuracy of notes taken and/or conclusions reached? Could we have added anything of value to their notes? If we raised questions during our conferences, what answers did someone promise to relay to us?

Advocating for Oneself at Care Conferences

Notes from the previous conference have not been reviewed before the newly scheduled conference to see whether any of my questions have been answered. For example, has my MDS State assessment identifier been changed to reflect my progress?

The rating speaks to the amount or kind of care a resident receives. It also affects the monthly cost a resident pays; the more care and equipment required, the higher the cost to the resident.

Throughout the long period of therapy, both at the facility and at CK, I've been identified as a MDS Case Mix Classification PC1 in the state's health care system. This means I have required much care and supervision at the facility, including using appropriate equipment for better and safer mobility. At all three of my past Care Conferences, I questioned why my rating had not changed to indicate all the progress I've made over all these months of therapy. Remember, I can even walk now with braces and a walker!

Yesterday (late August), I received a letter from the Health Department indicating a case mix classification notice with the same rating, PC1. I popped in to see the social worker. She sent a note to the nurse who does the classifications, and the nurse came to visit with me today. She asked me questions about my mobility and changed my classification to PB1. This is important because the cost of care is directly related to the classification assigned to each resident. Furthermore, my rating would be even higher if more staff were here to follow through continuously on the work done at CK. This work would enable me to make even more progress in mobility, thus earning an even higher rating, indicating little care is required.

All of the above have implications for how the state reimburses a facility.

Concern: New Glasses, A Saga

June 15, 2024

To: Billing Department, The Agency

Dear Ms. ---,

Below should serve as my response to your email of June 4 regarding account # ____. Please remember that when you make such policy decisions, you are affecting the lives of the elderly, many of whom cannot afford mistakes.

For your information, the contact I have spoken to several times about the eyeglasses is ---. I would have CC'd her, but did not have her email address.

Respectfully,
Sonja Schmieder

Good eyesight is essential for everyone. We all rely on our ability to see to help us achieve or maintain a high quality of life.

Vision changes are almost immediately noticeable to everyone but are especially noticeable as we age. We strain to see things near and far; we see things double. We dislike bright lights. Words in print need to be bigger, and reading anything becomes challenging. Driving at night is a real challenge.

We might need to work on getting our regular eye checkups that assess where we are on the need-for-glasses front or for any required adjustments to our present lenses. For sure, our eyesight worsens without proper care and accurate prescriptions.

I share with you here, then, an essential concern: the need for upgraded, accurately assessed glasses. It speaks to how problems are dealt with or not at nursing facilities and with their eye partner organizations. We know that Skilled Nursing Facilities work with outside service agencies to address some of the health needs of residents, including those about their eyesight.

This story also reminds us that we must be our own advocates when faced with an unjust situation. If we cannot advocate for ourselves, we are forced to rely on someone close to us to track and keep track of such affronts.

How many of us are visual learners? To see is to understand most things better. We can all agree on the importance of good eye care!

Management: Orchestrating Care

Several months ago, I noted that my progressive prescription of three to four years past was no longer as practical. Before approval to use MetroMobility, I took part in an on-site visit by an organization that works with my facility, conducting eyesight screening of residents. For a while, I wished to be well enough to visit my ophthalmologist and travel to his office more cheaply, using MetroMobility. This would take a bit of time, and as long as an eye doctor was conveniently on-site, I opted for an exam here.

Residents at the SNF should be forewarned about screenings. We also need to be apprised of the credentials and experience of doctors and assistants and the type of exams being conducted. No designated time is given for receiving new glasses. A facility worker tells us that screenings are taking place downstairs. You are on the list, and here we go!

According to its website, this group bills itself as a provider that helps "seniors in nursing homes and other long-term facilities get the unwavering support and healthcare they need." It offers diagnostic services and care for residents in podiatry, audiology, and optometry. Specifically, in optometry, this provider claims to deliver "detailed eye exams, visual field tests, eye pressure, and refraction tests." It also provides eyeglass prescriptions and "modifications to existing lenses."

For me, a detailed eye examination and selection of new frames at my facility resulted in a prescription forwarded to those at The Agency responsible for fulfilling it. The new glasses arrived at my facility a few weeks after the exam, following only one phone call to a representative at The Agency indicating a sense of urgency to receive them. I tried them on and realized, to my chagrin, that the new lenses could not be correct.

I called the representative there and told her about my disappointment with the new glasses, asking what I should do now. She said to wear them for a few weeks to allow my eyes to adjust. I tried to wear them but got too frustrated, knowing the glasses needed to be accurately assessed. I called her back; she said to mail them back to her, and she would have someone double-check them with what was prescribed. She called back a few days later to say that it was agreed that the glasses were incorrect and that she would have the factory make a brand-new pair, which she did.

Another few weeks passed. When the second pair of glasses arrived, I found they still needed to be corrected! I requested a refund of over $400 so that I could go to my own eye doctor. She said to return the glasses to her and contact their billing department to request a refund.

I gave the glasses to the person responsible for such mailings at my facility to mail back to The Agency. Unfortunately, they were not returned immediately and remained in the bookcase in her office for weeks. There is no sense of urgency here! The glasses were eventually returned to The Agency.

Another SNF resident broke his glasses. He asked daily when he would get new glasses as he did not have a backup pair. I can at least see some things with mine and still type missives on my phone! But who helps this man? Who advocates for him?

Management: Orchestrating Care

The Agency's Billing Department

After more weeks of waiting, I received an email from "billing." It read in part, *"We understand this may be disappointing news, and we apologize for any inconvenience this may cause... According to our policy, progressive glasses are non-refundable. As a result, we cannot issue a refund for your returned item."* (What? You call it "disappointing"? Outrageous, I say!)

Really? Now, I am not only out of the cost of the glasses, but I have also used my once-a-year exam, which is paid for by Medicare (as a social worker told me). If I go to my ophthalmologist now, I would have to pay for the exam and a new pair of glasses! However, with their expert care, I would most likely have no complaints about the final product!

All trust in this "pro-seniors" agency is gone! Will I take a chance on them a third time to make adjustments with the incorrect prescription? Would you? I will not. And I intend to call attention to those who make mistakes and expect the elderly to pay for them!

Like it or lump it? My course of action instead includes this email message and a phone message left with my County Ombudsman, the protector of resident rights! Copies of this concern were sent to management officials here. Some consideration was given to filing a formal grievance and sending copies to other interested individuals at agencies that address the mistreatment of elders!

The Agency "delivering the highest quality of healthcare" indeed!

Update: An email response from The Agency's Billing Manager (July 10, 2024)

"Hello Ms. Schmieder,

Please allow 2-3 business days for your refund of $411.27, which was refunded to the cc number ending in ---.

We value our patients and strive to maintain open communication and transparency. Please do not hesitate to contact us if you have any further concerns or require additional assistance."

Update 2:

I've just picked up my perfect new glasses from my optometrist's office. Good-to-go now!

For others who require screenings here, I suggest that residents be told beforehand what eye exams will be given and for what purposes. Residents should also know policies, including those for "returns." This way, they will be well-informed and not be left "blindsided."

Residents should also know how long it will take to receive their new glasses and any protocol for follow-up questions. These are only common courtesies that would be extended to those not in long-term care.

Concern: Discharge

In August, the then-acting Administrator and the head of the social work department hand-delivered me a letter notifying me that I would be discharged from this facility in a month for nonpayment of my debt, which is now in arrears. The letter stated that I would be discharged to another site (owned by the facility's parent company) and that I could file a written appeal of the proposed transfer to the state's Appeals Division.

I was stunned at how off-handedly they delivered such news to a senior resident, how quickly they left, and how they left the resident alone to deal with the news.

Filing An Appeal

I notified the Office of the Ombudsman for the County's long-term care services for assistance regarding this matter, as they frequently file appeals on behalf of residents in such facilities. I had the following questions about the discharge letter, which I shared with the Ombudsman and the social worker at CK, trusting in their advice.

- How can I confirm the accuracy of the amount owed, as my monthly statements indicate only a total amount due without any costs itemized or explained, e.g., the use of a Hoyer?

- How can I have a written plan for payment ready "upon receipt of this letter"?

- If I appeal this particular transfer within 30 days, how long will it take to make a decision before the discharge date?

- How does my pending MA application with the County affect that decision? A County Supervisor was to speak with me on Wednesday afternoon after 12:30 but did not call.

- Why choose a facility far from my immediate family and friends, including my grandchildren, who reside in the metro area?

- Why take me away from an area, the Twin Cities, where I have lived for 25 years? Is there no other facility that could accommodate my needs? What about my cancer doctors?

- How will I continue my rehabilitation work at Courage Kenny when I can't access transportation like MetroMobility?

- To which level of care would I be assigned: long-term (no longer needed) or assisted living?

- Cost?

- How will I reimburse this facility while paying for another accommodation?

- Is there some process of negotiation that now takes place with the facility?

- What kind of physical and occupational therapies are offered to residents there? How often?

- What means of transportation would I use to get to the new facility?

- Do I get in touch with the Ombudsman, or does someone else here?

I have never denied that I owe this facility for my time here and the services, care, and support I have received.

We filed an appeal of the discharge because of how the facility handled the proposed discharge. The facility needed to follow proper discharge procedures, including discussions with me before receipt of the letter and during the selection of a discharge site. Further, the Notice of Discharge was made while I still have an application for Medical Assistance pending.

Residents of SNFs do have rights!

As a result of our appeal, a preliminary hearing was conducted on August 14th by telephone with a judge assigned to the case. The Ombudsman represented me. The facility was represented by a law firm specializing in representing facilities in such cases and against residents.

Before the hearing, I requested information from the Ombudsman about preliminary hearings. I asked the following: Where will it be held via telephone? Who will be on the call? Is there a specific agenda for the hearing? Will I be asked questions, or will there be questions for the Ombudsman only? Remember that the other players in the scenario, namely residents, usually know very little about preliminary hearings.

The judge began by requesting which law applies to a nursing home discharge instead of a discharge from an assisted living facility, where the Judge believed I reside. Then, the judge asked some specific questions about me, including my age, how long I've lived at the facility, and whether my latest application for medical assistance is still pending with the state.

The judge asked the facility's lawyer, 'How did the facility get to this place of debt owed?' The judge inquired about their plan to call five witnesses, plus exhibits, for the regular hearing, saying, "How complicated is a nonpayment case going to be?"

The facility's lawyer requested more time than the customary two weeks after a preliminary hearing to prepare their case. After all parties consulted their calendars, the judge scheduled the regular hearing for September 4, in a month.

The judge recommended that we resolve the issue before the hearing. This means both sides negotiate and agree on a monthly payment to the facility.

A few weeks after the preliminary hearing call, the new administrator and a social worker visited my room to inform me that "in working with the Ombudsman and wanting to reach some resolution, the discharge notice issued to you … is hereby rescinded…. We intend to meet with you to further discuss a resolution and will set this up with you."

Upon their entering my room, I informed them that I had contracted COVID. They said they'd be in touch when I was feeling better. As I write this, my isolation period for COVID-19 has ended today. I will contact the Ombudsman for information on the meeting-to-be as I am more than ready for the prolonged nightmare to be over!

Update: Yesterday, I received a formal letter dated August 26, 2024, from the State of Minnesota, Office of Administrative Hearings for the Department of Health. It was an Order of Dismissal rescinding the Notice of Discharge, canceling any additional proceedings, and dismissing the case. The Ombudsman and I will continue discussing a repayment plan for this facility.

Update 2: The facility and I have agreed on a monthly repayment plan.

Concern: Availability of Water

Concern: There is always a suggestion that residents continue to drink lots of water lest they get dehydrated, especially during the warmer months. However, the nurses are the only ones dispensing water or monitoring its intake in conjunction with the disbursement of pills. Our trays include small glasses of ice water and juice, coffee, or tea, but we are frequently left with little or new fresh water. Note to aides: Please check if drinking water is available to each resident.

Concern: Showers

My once-a-week shower falls on Friday when my regular aide is off duty. For hours, I am left to guess who my aide is on the day shift and whether or not I will receive a shower, especially if the floor is short-staffed. Being a daily bather in real life, I am filled with angst, wondering what the story will be like from Friday to Friday. I find this unacceptable!

What is Plan B when someone does not make their shift, and the staff members who do show up for work are overwhelmed with too many residents on their lists to tend reasonably to anyone? They do their best to fill the void, but this unfair, unreasonable practice is becoming more commonplace.

The shower fiasco continues. Yesterday was Friday, the now infamous shower day, and the day when someone is assigned to help me with a shower, usually occurring on the day shift, between 9:30 and 2:30. I spoke with the aide around 7:00 am as we were getting me ready for a trip to the company that works with Courage Kenny on making and repairing braces; mine needed adjustments. The appointment was necessary, for I need braces or braces that work correctly to (yet) walk. I asked if I could have a shower around noon or later upon my return. I did not see my aide again, and no shower was given. During the night shift, I asked the nurse to please make a note that I had received no shower today, and he said he would.

So, today, Saturday, I talked with the nurse on duty to see whether I could get a shower. She said all aides already had their assignments for the day, so maybe on Monday. What?

A shower once every seven days is difficult to accept; extending that to ten days is absurd! She's working on it. But, who will the one assigned to help me in the shower resent more, the nurse giving her an added task, or the resident who would not settle for being told "Not today?"

One more thing relating to female residents: request that a note be posted to the chart of any female resident that female aides oversee any showers given. This does not necessarily have to do with any improprieties by male aides; I've never experienced or heard about any incident of impropriety here, but only the highest degree of professionalism and appropriateness practiced by each aide. The request speaks, instead, to a woman's (yes, even an old woman's) innate sense of modesty. By the way, my

Management: Orchestrating Care

husband felt the same way about female aides and their shower supervision.

Friday, December 6, 2024

Dear Management,

I wish to file a complaint (concern) that has to do with my latest shower debacle. Yesterday (shower day), my morning aide was getting me ready for my 5th cancer treatment session this week at the University. Since I expected to be back shortly after lunch, we agreed that she would give me a shower upon my return. She arrived in my room at 12:45 pm and asked if I was ready to go to the shower room.

Though tired from the week's treatments, I replied, "Yes!"

The aide said, "I'll be right back," and left the room. After 45 minutes of waiting for her to return, during which time Conrad came to take me for a walk, I decided that getting into bed for a rest was the better thing to do. I did not walk with Conrad, did not receive a shower, and slept for an hour and a half!

One of the aides on the afternoon shift volunteered to give me a shower after supper but got waylaid until 8:00 pm - too late to get into a shower. So, I asked the nurse to please leave a note for the am nurse to see if the schedule would allow someone (perhaps an aide with no showers to give on a Saturday morning) who would be willing to do so. I don't know that the note was delivered.

When the nurse came to give me my breakfast pills, I asked her if I would get a shower. She said that my aide for the day already had a shower to give and that maybe I could wait until Monday.

"No!"

Why? Because I am scheduled next week for the last five cancer treatments at the U and in the mornings. This means that I will not get back to the facility once again until after lunch and may not, once again, get my shower!

We hate to add to the day shift's schedule - giving residents showers is a production, as many of us are disabled and need extra help with our showers. It truly puts an added burden on the aides to do two showers on any shift, in addition to caring for all others' needs of those on their daily list. We discussed someone on the afternoon shift who might do so (preferably the aide from yesterday, who had volunteered to do so).

Update: The nurse returned and informed me that the aide on the day shift (today, Saturday) would shower me, adding another shower to her list of things to do. I am grateful but exhausted at having to address this whole shower thing each week. (Aren't you tired of listening to shower stories?)

Update 2: A New Year, An Old Shower Story. Friday was supposed to be my once-a-week shower day. Still, I had an MRI appointment followed by a couple of hours waiting for a doctor's appointment (totaling seven hours away from the facility). I didn't want to go with wet hair; I asked if someone on the evening shift could give me a shower or if any of the Saturday shifts could help. It's now Sunday, and after three days of being short-staffed on 2W, I still haven't received my shower.

Residents missing their showers face serious consequences. I have two appointments this week and fear I will have to go

Management: Orchestrating Care

stinky. Does the facility care that their residents might appear neglected by medical staff at hospitals and doctors' offices?

The nurses have requested additional staff support, but no managers are on duty because it is the weekend. What recourse do staff and residents have when there is seemingly no one in charge and limited monitoring or oversight at the facility? I've never heard of a nonprofit where the management team generally works 8:30–4:30, excluding weekends. Managing the care of over 100 elderly, sick, and disabled residents is a serious responsibility. It is not a job for "getting one's feet wet"; it requires a sincere commitment to the health and well-being of all residents. Far more than paperwork is needed to keep the operation running smoothly and maintain a good reputation.

Concern: Meds

My latest concern is one of my pills, the one that regulates hormones and affects metabolism. It is a pill dispensed at 4:00 or 4:30 am, often awakening me from a deep sleep, so a "no-show" is notable and noticeable, as I usually cannot fall back to sleep afterward.

For the past couple of weeks, I have not received a pill for several days in a row. I mentioned this to the nurse on the next shift and was told that they notified the pharmacy that I was out of that pill. At first, the pharmacy sent over five pills rather than the sheet containing pills to last for weeks. Once the five pills were used up, I again faced a couple more days without the pill.

Another nurse suggested that perhaps the follow-up fax requesting a refill of the prescription did not go through. He said he usually follows up the fax request with a phone call to the pharmacy, asking whether they received it. Not all nurses do that, or there is a problem at the pharmacy. At any rate, this is another reason for advocacy: the monitoring of meds.

I ask, "How are we residents expected to know about things to do with meds?" Trying to watch out for everything from meds to mice when feeling unwell is exhausting!

Concern: Autumn

Though we've had several evening sightings of mice in our room, no traps are set yet.

Concern: Fix it!

This facility is open 24 hours a day, seven days a week for residents, with security measures around the clock and designated hours for visitors. Like everywhere, the water is shut off for a while on some days, the main elevator doesn't work, and the TV goes blank. We can deal with it! That said, some things are unavailable to residents or not fixable "until Monday." This includes some necessary care supplies, some meds from the pharmacy (that usually delivers on a weekday schedule), the regulation of heat and air-conditioning, dealing with the sighting of a mouse (I do not sleep with mice!), an order for more peanut butter packets or Raisin Bran, a pen (a precious commodity), a broken window shade.

On weekends, nursing routines are disrupted when new or different staff take over or take on another shift. Regular staff members have to work some weekends as part of their job responsibilities. Activities are still offered on Saturday. Sundays are very quiet, even dull.

"'Cause there's somethin' in a Sunday makes a body feel alone."
Sunday Morning Coming Down by Kris Kristofferson

Concern: COVID Isolation

Residents should be told the projected date of their release from isolation so that they can reschedule any missed appointments. On the day of release, they should be included in a list of all those being released "first thing today" and notified of this.

Concern: Use of the Hoyer for Transport

The nurses' aides should have a plan for maneuvering the Hoyer to get a resident into a chair or wheelchair. This plan must be made before the resident is hoisted so that the resident will not be "in the air" in an uncomfortable sling that digs into sore and sensitive legs for even a short time. Aides should be mindful to avoid obstacles a resident's feet or legs may encounter while in transit, including the Hoyer itself.

Concern: Turning the Clock

Maintenance may plan to systematically turn the clocks in resident rooms back or forward, depending on the time of year. We residents must wait to have it done, sometimes for a week or more. Like most people, we "live by the clock" and do not appreciate not knowing the correct time.

Concern: Room Temperature

November 3, 2024

Dear Management,

It is unconscionable that residents and staff were expected to tolerate such high heat in residential areas over the past weekend with no recourse, even after multiple complaints about the situation!

Federal law requires facilities to be at "safe and comfortable temperatures" between 71 and 81 degrees Fahrenheit. No one from management or maintenance has come to measure the temperature in our respective rooms (and some rooms have no thermostat). However, good common sense will tell anyone that the temperature would have indicated (and still be at) over 81 degrees Fahrenheit.

What's wrong with that?

It's unhealthy, plain and simple! (A health concern for a health facility!). The elderly are at extremely high risk for stroke when room temperatures get too high, and many health conditions like diabetes and heart and kidney disease can be negatively affected by too high heat as well. Also, the staff are highly affected in their everyday routines, making them susceptible to ill effects.

For example, I've constantly had my fan going and the window wide open (though no air seemed to come in from outside); I've still felt nauseous. What about those residents whose rooms have no fans? (There's a fundraising idea!)

Management: Orchestrating Care

One person was told that the door (to the "furnace room," I assume) was locked, and nothing could or would be done until Monday. Is there no one from maintenance on call on weekends?

How can this be ignored? How much do we care about the health and well-being of our residents? Enough to control the temperature, which is controllable?

This is NOT an isolated incident. It has happened many times over the two winters I've spent here.

Sonja Schmieder

Concern: Mobility Care at the Facility & a CK Hiatus

Insurance dictates that only a limited number of therapy sessions are allowed within a specific time frame, even if the patient continues to make progress. I exceeded my limit at CK a few months ago and must now wait before I can return for sessions there.

In the meantime, when Conrad is on duty, I walk with him with braces for a few minutes every other day and every third weekend at the facility. That is not sufficient to have me walking by myself braces-free yet. (Or to enable me to "walk out of here!") As there presently is no one besides Conrad to help me, any real progress is stalled; I pray to retain/maintain what gains I have made.

It disappoints and frustrates me to have made such great advances at CK over six months and not to be able to build upon those advances here. This is once again a matter of a shortage of staff. At the very least, there should be a training session for the aides on working with the braces so that I can wear them daily (to stretch the muscles and keep the feet from contracting) when sitting in the wheelchair.

I look forward to resuming my therapy sessions at CK in the new year!

Update: Conrad will be getting additional help to walk residents.

Concern: Walking Daily

When my first course of therapy at Courage Kenny ended in early September, orders were given here to have staff put on my braces daily to continue to stretch my muscles and take daily walks. This was to include at least three trips with braces to the bathroom. I've walked only a handful of times in the past month due to sick staff, and the new trainee informed me that we would not be doing any walking because of the flu outbreak. I did not get my braces put on either (which I cannot do myself).

Because I walk so seldom these days, I am no longer good for anywhere near 200+ feet per walk. It's more like 50-100 feet at a time. I would have loved to walk with a mask, even though I've already had the nasty flu.

Concern: Where is Everyone?

> Saturday, December 21, 2024
>
> Dear Management,
>
> Over the past four months, I have noticed a marked difference in how care is delivered on 2West. I have been a resident at this facility for two years, and I find the changes in caregiving to be both

Management: Orchestrating Care

surprising and of concern. Here's what's happening (or not being attended to):

Residents' call lights are either not being answered or answered in a timely manner. This is important, particularly when the light is put on to request to go to the bathroom or to be changed so that a resident does not have to spend a long time in a soiled diaper; doing so causes rashes and chafing.

At the beginning of a shift, for the first couple of hours, there is no one (aides) to be seen. Not even in the halls. This means that residents themselves and/or fellow residents have to yell out for help. Where is everyone, and why is there not at least one person to keep track of the residents needing immediate attention? Someone should be named the designee to spot residents in trouble. Is this the job of the floater? And how many residents are on the floater's list? (Everyone on Floor 2?)

I've tried to answer my own question about the staff's whereabouts. Could they seem elusive because they are also expected to aid some residents on 2East as well? If so, I find that notion asking too much of those who already tend to several bedridden, disabled, and more difficult to tend to residents on 2West.

We also have had call-ins from staff members at the last minute to inform them that they will not be coming in to work their shift. Surprised? Why?

Spots are often not filled, then, and the work piles on for those who come to do their jobs - despite all that is put on them.

Retention and/or recruitment problems can start here.

Something is very wrong, and management needs to address it. The nurses and aides are not to be blamed for any of these shortcomings; they care about doing their jobs, and residents should not need to beg to be rightfully taken care of or tended to.

This is becoming a new normal and is simply not right. Moreover, it is correctable! Borrow people from other floors, hire more people, and provide staff with incentives for extra work.

Because of the staff shortage, resident diapers are often changed only once per shift. (It used to be two to three times per shift).

Once residents are put in their wheelchairs, there is a promise to return to make up their beds. It too often does not happen and is left as a chore for the next shift. This means residents' rooms look untidy throughout the day. Yes, that is unsettling and bothersome, especially when company visits.

Please consider these issues to be important ones.

Sincerely,

Sonja Schmieder

Concern: Illness

December 30, 2024

Dear Management,

This is a follow-up to the email I sent you on December 21, titled "Where Is Everyone?" — which has neither been responded to nor acknowledged. Please know that a few of us are still capable of pointing out what needs to be fixed or prevented and clearly outlining the best care and support all residents deserve. This should be the top priority for any facility and should never be ignored or lightly dismissed.

Late afternoon on Saturday (Dec. 28), I quite suddenly came down with a case of the flu.

After vomiting 20 times (Yes, I counted them, as it has been a while since this has happened - even beyond what I faced from chemotherapy treatments a few years ago), and adding to this was a not-so-nice case of diarrhea. Each time, it was my roommate who rushed to get help for me from the aide on duty, including a box to catch vomit and a change of clothes. (Not until she heard me and sought out help would anyone have checked and rechecked my status).

The night was uneventful; not during this time nor afterward did anyone take my temperature.

Around 4:30 am on Sunday, I asked if I could have a Ginger Ale and was told that the kitchen might have one but that I'd have to wait until breakfast (8:30). This was not what I wanted to hear, as I could tell I was dehydrated. I called my daughter, who eventually had some sent over, as well as Sprite and Gatorade.

I spent all day resting and did not get up to walk with Anne, Conrad's new assistant, who made sure that the kitchen eventually brought some Ginger Ale.

During the day, three full trays were brought in at mealtimes. Was there no communication with the kitchen on starting slow and small, with perhaps a piece of toast and some tea? Although I'm not sure I could have handled even that.

I understand that this is the holiday season and that there is little oversight of such happenings, but again, we are discussing people's well-being here.

Also, back to the overheating in rooms. My poinsettias have wilted from the heat in our room and a lack of watering. Sound petty? These were flowers given with love to create a festive Christmas atmosphere. And, to "roast" and be sick is asking a bit too much.

This flu seems particularly bad, and we need to be vigilant. We need to provide extra care to those dealing with yet another malady.

Sincerely,

Sonja Schmieder

Advocacy

You must be your own advocate. Admittedly, this depends on one's present state of health. This means taking the lead in your well-being and health, as well as that of the other residents. You know your needs and wants better than anyone else. Family and friends cannot always be there for you promptly; therefore, YOU must fight for your rights and the best care possible.

Nurses and aides are trained to sense when you might need or want something, but they are not mind readers. You need to say what you want and need, and you should do so nicely and firmly. This also applies to your communication with doctors. Ask questions, ask for help, and be direct and respectful.

Management: Orchestrating Care

You have the right to speak up. Ask about the plan for your health going forward. Ask about a timeline for reaching expectations. Pin him/her down!

Over the years, my friend Stan has had several relatives and friends residing in elderly care facilities. Before any move to such a facility, Stan recommends these two essential actions:

1. Choose a family member to serve as the designated advocate for the resident. (I'd add, even if the resident feels they can fend for themselves)

2. Have that person or the resident (if able) keep a diary with information and notations about the resident's daily routine, medications, hygiene matters, caretakers, meals, etc. (Once again, putting things in writing is hugely important.)

Stan reminds us that residents do have rights (he was an attorney!) and suggests that families become familiar with those rights before taking up residence at any facility.

Any facility should prominently display information regarding "patient" or "resident" rights. For this information, check out the Office of the Ombudsman at the State Department of Health.

For many months at the onset of GBS, I was incapable of advocating for anything or on behalf of anyone, especially myself. When you are very sick, your energy is concentrated on first surviving and, second, getting better, if even slightly better.

As residents make progress, the "fog of sickness" lifts.

Perhaps it lifts only a little at first, but enough that one begins to be aware of things happening—or not happening—around them. They sense that some things might need improving. They might notice the time it takes for a call light to be answered, the need to get something for pain "soon," a broken window shade that needs to be fixed, and pillows that need readjusting.

You suddenly want another cup of coffee, a radio to listen to music, a book to read, or a particular program to watch on TV. Then, you begin to have opinions and views about the goings-on, and you find your voice, even if it's loud; at this point, you may be self-advocating, which may even extend to making your own decisions about your health and well-being, in general.

This whole thing is, after all, about YOU. Be a leader, and take the lead on your own behalf. Advocate! Be concerned!

Conclusion

In any organization, there is room for error. Every place is flawed!

And so, I wrote about what things need fixing here. I sometimes voiced my concerns and suggestions for improvements, sharing them with those I trust and those who might take them seriously enough to incorporate them. Mostly, I write my ideas down so that I have a record of what I considered important at a specific time and why these things were important enough to me to pass along to those in positions of power.

These above-mentioned things needed attention! Fixing such usually requires a minimum amount of modification. Most problems do not require a new hire but only a rearrangement or restructuring of current management assignments geared toward overseeing such matters.

To residents: Feel free to put your concerns in writing! Perhaps receipt of such may not be adequately acknowledged courteously, but you will have a record of your notes and can refer to them repeatedly, if necessary.

My concerns each had their agony and ecstasy. Putting concerns in writing often requires reconstructing conversations and events; it can be laborious and time-consuming. However, the result can prompt positive action, which is the goal!

We can't just make noise! What we say has to offer something that will help move the needle forward and result in change for the good. We cannot only identify a problem (that's too easy); we must also present a solution.

Update: Management has acknowledged and addressed some of these concerns. Be a squeaky wheel!

Strength to Stand

5

Leadership in Action

The Minnesota Task Force on Aging

"The Legislative Task Force on Aging was established to review and develop state resources for an aging demographic; identify and prioritize necessary support for an aging population through statewide and local endeavors for people to remain in their communities; and ensure all age-related state policies are inclusive of race, gender, ethnicity, culture, sexual orientation, abilities, and other characteristics that reflect the full population of the state." (MN Laws 2023. Chapter 62, Article 2, Section 120)

The MN Task Force on Aging invited comments from the public about their mission and possible priorities. I provided the following written testimony to the members of the Task Force:

November 6, 2024

Madam Chair and Members of the Minnesota Task Force on Aging:

My name is Sonja Schmieder; I am 78 years old, an elderly person by all accounts, residing in a Skilled Nursing Facility (SNF) in Minneapolis.

I suffer from a rare neurological (not inherited or contagious) painful condition known as Guillain-Barré Syndrome (GBS), which affects the nerves and muscles and whose symptoms include numbness and tingling in the arms and legs, thereby impeding movement and mobility. This rapid onset-slow-to-recover disorder is the reason why I have spent almost two years in an SNF.

This means that I am not only an old individual but one who is infirm and disabled, as well. My experience- at one of many SNFs found throughout our state - has provided me with a bird's-eye view of resident life within this kind of "elderly housing" and of all who reside therein, which I now readily share with you.

I commend the State of Minnesota and the members of the Task Force for taking on this monumental responsibility, e.g., establishing a cabinet-level department, coordinating efforts of groups working on issues affecting the aging population, and providing increased funding for such efforts. Your findings -recommendations and decisions- could have wide-ranging, significant effects and impact on the aging population for decades to come.

A Consideration

It would behoove all of us—prior to making decisions about what must be done for our aging population—to demonstrate a thorough understanding of who are 'the aging.'. This includes not only statistical information about this fast-growing group but also accurate descriptions that avoid negative stereotypes, providing a more precise and comprehensive understanding of this target audience as people rather than simply as potential or current 'occupiers of beds' or individuals with diminishing faculties.

The following comments describe the aging population in Skilled Nursing Facilities and long-term care—focusing on the elderly and the oldest members of this group. This is a plea for a deeper understanding of who we truly are.

Long-Term Care Residents

Even though we are elderly and facing health challenges, we still cherish our families and friends, fond memories, a good idea, a good joke, and the thrill of a well-laid plan—one that might just spark a bit of mischief!

Contrary to popular belief (or gross exaggeration), most of us are not going to drop dead in the next five minutes or even for years yet!

We are not nearly as active, vigorous, enthusiastic, or "fresh" as we once were; we are, instead, knowledgeable, experienced, and seasoned.

We feel sad and bad that what you see is not who we are, nor who we were "back then," when we could add value, when we thought we really mattered, and when we looked good.

We mourn the loss of our independence. We long for some privacy.

We do not like being invisible to most people. We hate being ignored or, worse, avoided.

We don't want to be excluded or isolated from most things; we experience a fear of missing out (FOMO).

We do not appreciate our awkwardness, our inelegance. We are self-conscious about any impairment. We think we must look funny, and that is not okay.

We do not handle our failing eyesight well or having to say, "Pardon me. What did you say?" repeatedly.

No matter our condition, we fight to survive, to stay alive—just like a sick puppy or leaves wilting on a tree.

Most of us believe in God and trust in prayer.

At this stage in our lives, we've stopped caring about accumulating 'things,' making it 'big' in our careers, being liked by everyone, or being the best at anything—except Bingo!

We care that our bodies are clean, our minds able to function, and our words readily available.

At times, we (still) long to go home, attend a regular church service, drive our own car, take part in community activities, meet someone for happy hour, attend a really important family event, or have an intellectual, even argumentative, discussion.

We believe there is value and worth in work; we miss terribly our respective worlds of work.

We cherish our nurses—our comforters and cheerleaders.

We continue to make new friends.

We care that everyone practices good manners and shows respect for each other. (We demanded that of our children).

We have a strong sense of fairness and justice: what's right is right, and in the end, it is right that always wins. (We told our children that.)

We honor our civic duty; we respect the rule of law, pay our taxes, and vote.

We notice and care when things are not well-planned or nicely coordinated, but we do not want to be in charge of anything!

Even now, we like to learn, and we still enjoy a gifted teacher.

We care that someone reaches out to us. Or for us.

There are days, or just (powerful) moments, when we feel we need to "go back" in time; we have trouble accepting that we cannot do so.

Ever optimistic, we look to the future. As we always have.

We can shift the conversation about older adults from the common, often negative perceptions of them as sick, feeble, slow, tired, or lonely—though some of these words may apply—to more hopeful language that highlights their knowledge, wisdom, insight, sensibility, experience, courage, determination, decisiveness, cleverness, and the richness of their lives.

Can you imagine how an emphasis on the positivity of the aging adult could affect the self-image and esteem of this group of individuals, as well as their emotional and physical health? Can you even guess how uplifting a message you would send to those who might be written off, discarded, or abandoned as hopeless or just "marking time?"

You have the power to positively transform the perception of aging in Minnesota—through the attitudes you adopt and the words you choose to define these individuals.

Thank you.

Sonja Schmieder

Leadership of SNFs

This brings me to my obsession (yes, that is what it is) with leadership or a lack thereof. The healthcare system at all levels needs high-quality leadership. It must be assessed, revamped, aligned, updated, redesigned, and reworked, and the good pieces must be built upon.

Yes, this can be done. In addition to the MN Task Force on Aging, a small select group of thought leaders in healthcare could do the following: paint a big picture of where we now are, point out gaps and flaws that need to be addressed, divide the big picture into themes and topics, select more leaders (and scholars) to convene other experts to address the issues, gather pertinent info and analyze it, decide where we should go with it, set tasks, write up reports, share results, ask for feedback, do the required PR to get everyone on board, create a final version, disseminate it and go with it. It has been done before!

We need to advocate for everyone's healthcare and for a friendlier, more effective system that is easy to navigate and works for everyone. We need to fight for an efficient and effective system that gives equal billing to the elderly and infirm.

Leaders, come together to take this on! As our population lives longer, everyone must care about creating and enforcing the best healthcare system imaginable. Let's choose our leaders and choose them wisely.

For years, leadership has fascinated me because the success or failure of any endeavor depends upon the upfront, effective, and honest actions of individuals we call leaders.

I want the strongest leaders in our Skilled Nursing Facilities! We need those with vision, emotional intelligence, compassion, and conviction to tackle and streamline the healthcare system's vagaries. We need those who can provide guidance and orchestrate reform.

Ask, "Is the entity successful?" Look to its leadership for the answer.

Leadership: What It Means

No matter the mission of an organization, the initiative, or the program, a leader will pour everything they have into leading and presiding over it. The charge is all important and all-consuming. A leader makes it happen by "wearing the cause" and wanting something positive to happen!

- Leaders beget leaders; strong leadership on the Board bodes well for filling other key organizational positions with other effective leaders.
- "Leadership is action!" (Allen Schmieder)
- Most leaders dare to think and act "outside the box"; they do so naturally and instinctively.
- Leaders demand more of themselves and others.

Leadership: Why the Fascination?

The most successful SNFs will have the most effective leaders in the long run.

Leaders go beyond focusing on a piece of a puzzle or a single undertaking; they look beyond their immediate responsibilities. Leaders concentrate on the puzzle itself. Their broad, big-picture view of the organization brings its mission and goals to life. It prompts the need for a deep understanding of the people involved and their interactions with them at all levels. This focus on the entirety and success of the enterprise, including all departments such as finance, admissions, and Human Resources, allows leaders to view the organization from multiple perspectives and as a whole.

- Leaders are a select and rare group of individuals who do much more than manage people and things.

- Leaders create a strong and workable vision for the organization. They talk about the vision a lot so everyone associated with the organization is on the same page.

- Leaders have the status of being the most effective and visible communicators in the organization. They build up the organization's credibility with intelligence, expertise, honesty, creativity, patience, and persuasion. They fearlessly take calculable risks. They network; you never know who might have a good idea for you.

- Leaders set the pace for the organization and go the distance, no matter the many obstacles they face. They are intelligent people who problem-solve and create solutions with self-confidence. They foster new ideas and opportunities for employees to grow personally and professionally.

- Leaders treat people with respect, courtesy, and kindness, which benefits them and their respective causes tenfold! This fosters loyalty and productivity.
- They know instinctively that what they do is good and right for the organization. They create fine-tuned machines that run well and make things work better. And they raise the morale of everyone.
- They make it all look so easy.

The leaders I have known are fearless in their creativity and adjusting the rules when the situation demands it. They find better, more effective ways to succeed beyond what the rules dictate while keeping their defining principles intact.

Leaders find ways for management and staff members to grow through training experiences and other learning opportunities.

This facility was established in 1946, and someone led its founding. And, in its continuance! I just cannot, however, yet feel the pull, the magnetism a leader exudes where you know someone is in charge, in control, and going somewhere!

Fostering New Leadership

There are those at this facility who are certainly capable of leading and have the potential to be fine leaders. It requires these individuals to want to step up to the occasion and step it up a notch from where they presently find themselves.

Note: There is a marked difference between leading a facility and "taking the lead" in various ways when doing one's job.

The new administrator here has just begun acclimating to the position. Go forth and lead!

What Leadership Is Not

You now have a picture of what I think defines effective leadership. Here are a few thoughts about what is not selfless nonprofit leadership. This is not a definitive list by any means.

Leadership is not:

- Just good management
- A title, a particular office setting, a huge salary, or perks offered
- About who wields the most power
- Thinking that being a part of an establishment with a good reputation is good enough

Leadership is not:

- Ignoring that a leader is still part of a team and should first address the needs and wants of the organization's members, residents, customers, or clients
- Comprised of random undertakings that may or may not have anything to do with the facility's mission

- About putting on a show or making a loud noise without pressing a coherent plan of action for success

Leadership does not:

- Promote a personal agenda rather than an organizational one, nor is it about personal gain over gains made for the organization to continue its work

Some Real Leaders

Upon graduation from the University many years ago, I became a member of the teaching profession. Although my students were my passion and the primary focus of my time and energy, I also became an active participant in professional activities. At the state association level, I served on committees, made presentations, and wrote reports and papers on timely issues primarily related to instruction and professional development.

As my interest grew in association work, I became the Association's representative to several statewide Department of Education committees. For example, I helped develop Continuing Education Requirements for the Recertification of Teachers and A Code of Ethics for the Teaching Profession in Minnesota. This work led me to serve on several National Education Association (NEA) committees.

Eventually, I went to work full-time at the NEA in Washington, DC. This work opened up a whole new world to me, expanding my knowledge base in the field of education and my network of colleagues across the nation, although this did not happen quickly or naturally.

I was a young teacher from a small town who found herself in circumstances she had never imagined. I doubted my ability to rise to expectations and represent fellow teachers honestly and fairly. I looked for leaders and women role models, especially, and found two. Though this was 50 years ago, I still remember their effect on me.

One was Eva Baker, a California-based educational researcher whose areas of expertise were accountability, assessment, testing, and evaluation. Heavy! She just marched to that podium with confidence and belief in her data and scientific conclusions and delivered her papers to an international conference of participants. She was accepted as an equal, lauded, and admired for her work and presentation. How did she do that? I wanted to do that, too, and be like her. Almost 20 years later, at another conference, I met her and told her about that consequential day.

My second role model was Joan Growe, Minnesota's former Secretary of State. She knew her job, took the lead, and worked tirelessly on voter registration, rights, and participation issues. She always conducted herself with grace, courage, and humility.

Both women chose their niche, opted for the stage, and changed the game. Not much was allowed to get in their way. That's leadership! Our representation of women as inspirational leaders still needs to be more prolific. But things are changing!

Please note that I am aware that countless women do their jobs well. Who often serve as "the wind beneath [our] wings." My mom was one of those women who kept everything together so that the rest of us could fly! She didn't choose to be a leader.

Leadership in Action

How many of our Skilled Nursing Facilities have leaders at the helm?

We sorely need visionary and strategic leadership at all levels of society, especially in the healthcare sector. Strong and effective leaders are required to meaningfully address the care and support of the elderly, particularly those in long-term care.

The following passages describe a few leaders I know or have known. I point out some of their leadership attributes and indicate how they have taken the lead in significant accomplishments.

Extraordinary Leaders in the Field of Education and Other Areas

My husband, Allen, was a distinguished geography professor at the University of Maryland and the Ohio State University. He was also a charismatic leader, inspirational speaker, and giant and pioneer in educational reform and improvement at the national level for decades at the U.S. Department of Education in Washington, DC. He knew the way to go, saw what needed to be done, and did it. He loved life and people. To him, nothing was impossible.

> *"And if I listen to my heart, I'll hear your laughter once more."*
> *"Goodbye" sung by Kenny Rogers*

My father, Mathew, was a community icon who dared to dream of and organize an American Legion World Series baseball tournament in a small town in northeastern Minnesota. He moved people and things! He also cared deeply about veterans, especially those who might be in need or simply "lost."

My mom used to say, "You are known by the company you keep."

My closest friends include those in their 70s and 80s, who continue to lead to this day and share their ideas and opinions on what requires action. I feel fortunate to learn from them or just be in the same room with them! They offer solutions to problems and provide never-ending energy to their respective broad-based initiatives. They build things and then leave them in capable hands.

My friend Greg has degrees in dentistry and pathology. He had a stellar 15-year career as a medical researcher at the National Institutes of Health (NIH) and Johns Hopkins University investigating Respiratory Syncytial Virus (RSV), a common respiratory virus with a name that is now familiar to us all. He was the CEO of a biotechnology company in Maryland and is now the CEO of a biological research laboratory in Utah that focuses on diagnostic and testing solutions for patient care. He is a businessman, author, and historian of the Church of Latter-Day Saints.

On a recent birthday of his, I wrote:

> *"It all begins at an early age: something inside certain people begs for more. They see a bigger picture beyond their very cozy and comfortable world. This knowing produces an idea that defines some important and unmet needs. It won't let go! So, these individuals "take action." They go about doing something about it!*
>
> *The "something" speaks loudly to like-minded others and is not deterred by those who cannot "get it!"*

We call such extraordinary people "leaders" (not to be confused with most individuals in any leadership position). Leaders know how to get things done! They have a heart and a reliable sense of direction and are adept at following through. They possess vast amounts of integrity, decency, courage, energy (zest), empathy, and persistence.

There is no pause, no rest! Over time, for many of these people, the cycle of "taking the lead" must repeat itself, and often, many times.

I wish an exceptionally fine leader an extra-special and happy birthday filled with endless cycles of moving and implementing great ideas, with tons of know-how, patience, and courage."

Sonja

Greg's wife, Jalynn, is a philanthropist, photographer, and a Founder of Madison House Autism Foundation in Rockville, Maryland. Another impressive leader!

After meeting an outstanding individual's spouse or significant other, my husband and I would remark that we now have a twofer to help aid in whatever cause we were involved in. Bright meets bright = a powerful force for good!

My Friend Rick

Inventive, imaginative, ingenious Rick is a former astronaut and chief scientist at NASA's Marshall Space Flight Center in Huntsville, AL. He was a Physics Professor and a Science Communications Lecturer at Vanderbilt University. He is currently working as a member of the Marshall Retirees Association to raise funds to build a NASA Space Exploration

Wall of Honor to recognize those in Huntsville and their families who made space exploration possible.

He is a warm-hearted, kind, and gentle gentleman. Rick and my husband, Allen, were detailed from their regular jobs for a year to help start and coordinate VP Al Gore's White House GLOBE Initiative. GLOBE stands for Global Learning and Observations to Benefit the Environment and is a hands-on science and education program, now in over 100 countries. In a note to our friend, Rick, I praised his leadership: "You see it (whatever needs to be done), most can't; you act (to change it), most won't; you achieve (success) when few do; and, then you move on – to another 'promise' (challenge)."

A Top-notch Lawyer

If you wanted to take your great idea (the likes of which no one has ever heard of!) to a higher, more widespread, yet protected level, why, you'd run to my friend Stan! In 1968, Stan and two other young attorneys in their mid-twenties founded a patents and trademarks law firm in the Washington, DC area. They located their firm near the U.S. Patent & Trade Office. They aimed to protect their clients' good ideas, inventions, and intellectual property. Their success led to a partnership with a Japanese patent law firm in Tokyo, where I worked briefly.

This partnership was the first of its kind. To me, Stan was the one who kept the firm au courant and on the cutting edge, especially at the onset of the technology revolution with its many processes and innovations that needed patent protection. He was the visionary, the risk-taker, the one who pushed the boundaries of opportunity. Years ago, the law firm made room for the next generation of leadership; today, it is one of the nation's largest and most prestigious firms.

Three Minnesota Education Leaders

Tom, Bob, and Rick K. are three people who made enormous contributions to the education of children and youth, to the teachers with whom they worked in their respective communities, and to the education community at large.

Tom is a retired school principal whose strong leadership, confidence, and style of persuasion helped design and build the avant-garde, technology-centered, technology-rich Eagan High School.

Bob, a former K-6 teacher and principal, was a team member of one of the first open classrooms in Minnesota. He has been an active member of his community's Lions Club, spearheading educational proposals and programs. Bob's leadership style is empowering others, motivating and encouraging them to make independent decisions, and achieving things they may have thought impossible. Bob is the quintessential professional and community representative.

I met my friend Rick K. many years ago when we, both Minnesotans, participated in the National Education Association's (NEA) Teacher Center Project, a unique, federally funded staff development program for teachers. Rick was a Teacher Center Director at one of 48 NEA sites across the country; each center elected its director from the ranks of teachers in its respective district.

This experience involved teachers taking the lead, designing their professional development programs, and serving on their policy boards. He says it was a launching point for a career that included serving as a state representative for 12 years, Speaker Pro Tempore of the Minnesota House of Representatives, President of the Minnesota High Tech Association (MHTA), and Executive Director of the Minnesota Transportation Alliance.

All three leaders are highly respected and loved by their fellow educators and communities.

To the Minnesota Task Force on Aging:

All of the leaders mentioned above prioritize people over policy and plans of action and have proven track records. Look for this kind of leader as you dictate the changing face of aging in our state. Without strong leadership, having your new vision taken seriously or thriving will be almost impossible.

"The wisdom of the owl is a guide for those who seek the truth." Unknown

Gaining an Understanding

If you've reached this point in reading this book, you may think, "I had no idea!" Remember what Keats said, "Nothing ever becomes real until it is experienced."

Here's what I think we've become aware of:

We learned about the residents in long-term care and their ongoing need for support.

Being in long-term care causes residents to have to make huge adjustments to their thinking and in their goals and plans.

How difficult that can be for residents to accept.

Long-term residents' bodies and sometimes even their minds are failing, but they still feel, think, and fight to survive.

How important it is for residents to maintain their dignity.

Ways we rely on the good will of others for care and support.

How dearly residents value ongoing interactions with family, friends, the nursing staff, physical and occupational therapists, social workers, and those in management. How grateful residents are for their attention and support, their thoughts and prayers.

How crucial to maintaining positive mental health are human connections, activities, exercise, sleep, faith, and the sure knowledge that each resident is (still) wanted, needed, and prized.

What it takes to run a Skilled Nursing Facility, and the critical role outstanding leadership and sound management practices play in its success.

Matters of Concern that will arise at any facility.

The solace, strength, and comfort residents appreciate when facilities address residents' concerns.

The role of residents as advocates in their own health and well-being.

Guillain-Barre Syndrome and a need for more research to ease the symptoms of this rare neurological condition and help prolong life.

There is more! But I will leave you now with these things to consider: what it is like to be a resident of a Skilled Nursing Facility and how an insider's perspective might more accurately identify residents' critical issues and concerns, and articulate ways a facility might address them.

Thanks for reading! I hope you learned a lot about long-term residents and their lives in long-term care.

> *"Nothing in life is to be feared. It is only to be understood. Now is the time to understand more, so that we may fear less."*
> *Marie Curie*

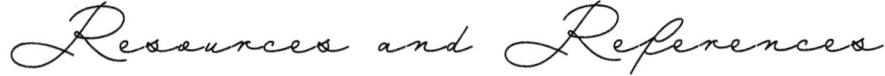

Resources and References

Allina Health: Guillain-Barré Syndrome (GBS) Service Line. Retrieved from https://account.allinahealth.org/servicelines/815

American Psychological Association. (n.d.). *Mental health*. Retrieved from https://www.apa.org/topics/mental-health

Centers for Disease Control and Prevention. (2022, October 19). *Mental health*. Centers for Disease Control and Prevention. https://www.cdc.gov/mentalhealth/

Mayo Clinic. (n.d.). *Guillain-Barré syndrome (GBS)*. Mayo Clinic. Retrieved from https://www.mayoclinic.org

Minnesota Department of Human Services: Explore resources and information on services provided by DHS, supporting the well-being of Minnesota residents. Visit https://mn.gov/dhs/.

Minnesota Nursing Home Report Card: Provides details about nursing home options, including star ratings for "resident quality of life, family satisfaction, and inspection results." Available at nhreportcard@dhs.mn.gov.

National Institute of Allergy and Infectious Diseases (NIAID). Retrieved from https://www.niaid.nih.gov/

U.S. Department of Health & Human Services. (n.d.). *Health Insurance Portability and Accountability Act (HIPAA)*. Retrieved from https://www.hhs.gov/hipaa"

Strength to Stand

About The Author

Following brain surgery, radiation, and chemotherapy treatments, Sonja Stukel Schmieder contracted Guillain-Barré Syndrome (GBS), a rare neurological condition. This led to hospital stays and tryouts at more than a few Skilled Nursing Facilities in the Twin Cities. She has remained at one of them in long-term care for 22+ months and counting. She prompts a fuller understanding of the residents and their lives inside such facilities from an insider's point of view. She goes beyond a brief study to a complete examination of this kind of organization to help readers get a more accurate picture of the workings of such facilities.

Sonja is passionate about sharing her experience to foster understanding and compassion for those living in long-term care. As an educator at heart, she is available to speak with groups interested in learning more about life inside these facilities and the challenges faced by residents. For speaking engagements or inquiries, please contact her at sonjaschmieder3737@gmail.com.

www.ingramcontent.com/pod-product-compliance
Lightning Source LLC
Chambersburg PA
CBHW070625030426
42337CB00020B/3922